Warning

Do <u>not</u> abruptly stop taking your medication since this is very dangerous. Only do this gradually under the guidance of a knowledgeable doctor.

Table of content

Preface

This book was written to protect primarily our children's physical and mental health and also to protect the public from irrational killings and mass killings. It urges parents, caregivers, teachers, doctors, healthcare providers, politicians, judges and other members of the legal system to become informed about the dangers of psychiatric drugs and to make the right moral decisions.

I do not intend to criticize the many wonderful caring doctors and professionals, who would be surprised to learn of the dangers involved in these drugs.

And I want to thank all the authors whom I listed and quoted who were courageous and critical and who spent so much of their time doing research on these psychotropic drugs and who probably, to some extent, risked their careers doing this. It would have been easier to just acquiesce.

I want to especially thank Dr. Peter Breggin, the "conscience of psychiatry" as he is called, who has devoted his life to help humankind with their battle with psychotropic drugs. He has researched a huge amount of material to prove the drugs' dangers. All of his invaluable books should be required reading.

And finally, I want to thank William Campbell, who helped me, as always, with his support on the computer to create this book.

*

(I have added my own comments in parenthesis and I have emphasized (underlined) what I thought was important. The statements of some authors were repeated by other authors. I usually left these because of their importance.

All references to the "Tribune Review" means the "Tribune Review" published in Greensburg, PA.

I also want to add that I am not a scientist, just a teacher and parent, and that I am very concerned about this issue and that I want to inform the public about these dangerous drugs.)

The most important part of our body is the brain. It is a mixture of chemical and physical actions and reactions which we are far from understanding. It is also the seat of knowledge, creativity, conscience, courage, righteousness.

Let us protect the brain and keep monetary forces from damaging it with psychiatric drugs, especially since we don't know what the far-reaching consequences of taking these drugs are.

"He loved the truth for truth's sake, and for man's sake." *

*Robert Ingersoll about Thomas Paine, quoted in Levine, Bruce, p.25

1. Introduction

I first encountered psychiatric drugs when a teacher recommended putting one of my children on Ritalin. This child was in middle school and had a tendency to forget his/her pencil. He/she also was a good student and a lively and curious child. I researched the medication and read – to my horror – what the side effects were: stunted growth (but not more than a few inches, as one counselor advised me), damage to the heart, depression, even suicidal thoughts and actions. All this, just to ensure more compliance of a healthy, lively 12-year-old? (Experts tell us now that sitting for seven hours isn't exactly healthy for a growing child.) I called two pediatricians, one a very trusted one in the community, the other one my sister- in- law, and asked for advice. They assured me that the medication was safe. After seeing my child become paler and nervous, I decided to take the recommended dose (three tablets a day at 5 mg) myself. It was like having drunk ten cups of coffee. (Interestingly, my friends were shocked about this – this proves the deep seated (and false) assumption that the diagnosis of ADHD proves that there are some chemicals missing in the brain and that Ritalin would correct this problem and they felt that since I didn't miss that chemical, something dreadful would happen to me. Strangely, they thought that I had a lot of courage doing this.)

This incident caused me to become suspicious of psychotropic drugs. I collected many articles about crimes that stated that the murderer or the person who had committed suicide had been under psychiatric care. In the beginning the drugs taken were mentioned by name. This is rarely the case now.

I believe that the public misjudges the mental health crisis. They do not see that psychotropic drugs (often in conjunction with guns) cause many earthshattering crimes like school shootings. As a judge recently stated about a case he was involved in (the murderess had killed her cousin with whom she was on friendly terms, had been diagnosed with mental illness at 12 and had been prescribed as many as 10 medications - she also used marijuana): "It's such a sad case, and it was so unnecessary… It was such a bizarre act in this case, such an unexplainable result, and it's difficult for me to understand." (Tribune Review, April 26, 2022).

Many people see the chemistry involved in the structure of these drugs as too difficult to understand. They believe those who claim that mental illness is hereditary or a sign of a chemical imbalance. Unfortunately, even the scientists who work for the NIH (National Institute for Health, a government entity) claim this. They write: "Scientists understand that mental illnesses are associated with changes in neurochemicals." (NIH. National Library of Medicine/2007 Bookshelf ID: NBK 20369) People in general don't know what bipolar, clinical, psychotic or schizophrenia really means (the experts themselves often have a hard time to definitively characterize these disorders!) but are impressed by those terms. They are taken in by commercials. They sometimes think that their lot in life is just too hard and that they need drugs to help them cope. They often don't read the important books about this topic or inform themselves about the side effects of the drugs. They often simply don't have or take the time.

In writing this book I am trying to give an overview of criminal cases involving psychotropic drugs, to help the lay person to understand the chemistry and the financial background that explains their popularity, the many problems with these drugs and their use and possible solutions or – at least, small steps that could be taken to alleviate these problems.

I have written a short book – (many great books have been written about this topic – see bibliography at the end of this book)–so that it may help individuals, parents, teachers, persons in the medical field and judicial arena to form an independent opinion and act courageously in this matter.

These are just some cases, there are many more that appear daily in the papers. I did not include those that do not mention mental illness and treatment, although those might be involved in many more cases.

I quoted the sources that refer to the use of psychotropic drugs, most often Wikipedia, because this website lists most sources referring to the individual cases. I accessed all the Wikipedia information in this matter on April 25, 2024.

Aiello, Sydney, 19, Parkland, FL. (s. Cruz, Nikolas), victim. She was a Parkland shooting survivor who shot herself a year after the Parkland shooting. (NBC news, March 22, 2019) According to the Washington Post, Sydney had been diagnosed with PTSD and had been treated for it. There was another victim in the aftermath of the Parkland shooting who committed suicide, but her name is not known. (Washington Post, March 25, 2019)

Alexis, Aaron, Navy Yard shooter, killed 12 people, had been treated for various mental health issues (Time, Sept. 17, 2013), according to Wikipedia, with Trazodone.

Allen, Christina, drowned her three- year- old son. "Her mother has said that she was on medication for nerves." (Las Vegas world news, posted March 10, 2014)

Allen, Christine, Canada. She was charged with two counts of aggravated assault and administering a noxious substance after two children in her care were hospitalized. (She put eye drops into the children's juices in the daycare center she ran.) "Her claim (in court?) also stated that she suffers from psychological issues - including anxiety, depression and bipolar disorder- for which she claimed to take medication regularly." (Toronto Star, July 23, 2013)

Bowers, Robert, committed the Pittsburgh Synagogue shootings on Oct.27, 2018. He had a mental health history and had been treated with Effexor, (according to the Trib. Review, July 21, 2023)

Card, Robert. He killed 18 people in Maine. "He struggled with mental health issues in recent months" (Tribune Review, Oct.27, 2023)

Carter, Aaron, of the Backstreet Boys, may have died of suicide. "he had been open about his struggles with substance abuse as well as various mental health conditions…he repeatedly checked into Rehab." (Los Angeles Times, cited in the Tribune Review, Greensburg, Nov. 7. 2022.) "Cans of compressed air were found in his bedroom…along with prescription pills" (Celebrity News, Nov.8, 2022) According to Wikipedia, he drowned after he took difluoroethane (a gas) and alprazolam. (Xanax).

Croft, Ashley, 38, of Vandergrift, PA., killed her cousin John Edward Smail of Greensburg in 2018. There was no animosity toward him. Her defense attorney, Patrick Thomassey, stated : "She was diagnosed with mental illness at twelve and had been prescribed as many as ten medications." (Trib. Review, April 26, 2022)

Crumbley, Ethan, 15. He killed four students at his Michigan high school in 2021. "The shooter… has major depression, anxiety and obsessive –compulsive disorder" according to his psychologist. (Associated Press (AP), in Trib. Review, August 2, 2023)

Crusius, Patrick. He killed 23 people in El Paso. His attorney said: "He suffers from severe mental illness". (The week, July 21, 2023)

Cruz, Nikolas, Parkland, Fl. In February 2018 he killed 17 people. He was put into an orphanage after birth and then was adopted. Both of adoptive parents died. He was orphaned three months before the shooting. He was diagnosed with ADHD and ODD (Oppositional Defiant Disorder) and Depression "for which he took medication." (Sun Sentinel, Feb. 24, 2018).

Denison, Debra, shot two of her grandsons and herself on February 28, 2013 in Preston, CT. She had attempted suicide before and had been committed. A relative is quoted as saying "When she would be depressed, she would be running to the doctor getting prescriptions." (Daily Mail, Feb. 28, 2013)

Foss-Greenaway, Brooklyn, three- month old victim, 2012. She was killed by a ten–year-old, Kelly Murphy, who had been treated for behavioral disorder. Foss had traces of Murphy's ADHD medication in her system. (AP, cited in the Tribune Review, October 23, 2012)

Flanagan, Sharon, drowned her two-year old son in a Greentree hotel in Allegheny County. Her husband stated: "I tried to commit her for a second time." (KDKA, Dec.9, 2012)

Gendron, Payton, 18, killed 10 African American people in Buffalo, New York. "He occasionally licked and clenched his lips "(a sign of side effects of psychotropic drugs?) during his trial. He had had a "mental health evaluation that put him in a hospital for a day and a half" ((AP) cited in Tribune Review, Nov. 29, 2022)

Green, Dayvon, Maurice, College Park, Maryland, a graduate student, killed his roommate and himself. "[He] had been prescribed medication." (Tribune Review, February 13, 2013)

Hadley, Tyler, 17, killed his parents with a hammer on July 16, 2011. He had taken 3 pills of Ecstasy before, but he also had taken the antidepressant Citalopram (Celexa) "Evidence hints at some mental problem…. Including a receipt from a mental health Center and a bottle of Citalopram, an antidepressant." (abc 25 WPBF News)

Harris, Eric and Klebold, Dylon, 18 and 17 (Columbine shooting), Colorado, April 20, 1999. They died of self- inflicted wounds. According to Wikipedia, in 1998 they broke into a locked van to steal computers and other items. They were charged and offered to have their record expunged if they agreed to psychiatric treatment. "Harris wanted to join the United States Marine Corps but…was rejected shortly before the shooting because he was taking Fluvoxamine (Luvox) which he was required to take as part of court ordered management therapy."

(The families of five Columbine high school shooting victims were suing the maker of the antidepressant Luvox by Solvay. In the law suit it was claimed that Solvay failed to warn Harris' doctor about the side effects. "Such drugs caused Eric Harris to become manic and psychotic." (AP cited in Trib. Review, no date avail.)

Hartmann, Brynn, killed her husband, comedian Phil Hartmann, and herself. According to the "Los Angeles Times"(May,1999) she had used Zoloft.

Hinckley, John W. He tried to assassinate President Roald Reagan. "Dr. David Barr of the Harvard Medical School, a defense psychiatrist…: " prescriptions for the tranquilizer Valium and an antidepressant drug were found in the hotel room where Hinckley stayed before the shooting." (upi.com (https://www.upi.com1982/05/18))

Hromanic, Michael, victim, died after he had taken an MAOI, an antidepressant. Hypertension is a known side effect. He died of a stroke. (Trib. Review, August 30, 2020)

Kasantsev, Artiom, Russia. He killed seventeen students and wounded 24, before he committed suicide. He had been "a patient at a psychiatric facility." (AP, Tribune Review, Sept.27, 2022)

Keepers, Natalie, Virginia Tech. In January 2016 she was an accomplice in killing a thirteen - year old whom she had never met. "She harbored suicidal thoughts in middle school. She learned to cope through therapy and medication in high school" (Washington Post, cited in Trib. Review, no date avail.) A psychiatrist was quoted as saying that she had been diagnosed with six mental disorders. (10news, Sept. 20, 2018)

Kinkle, Kip. He was fifteen, when he killed his parents and two students. "Expert testified that he was psychotic ...and deeply depressed." "According to a friend... Kip had just been put on Prozac ...Prozac has been claimed as a mitigating factor in criminal cases so many times," (Huffington Press, June 20, 1998), (Trib. Review, June 20, 1998 and Nov. 11, 1999.)

Kreutzer, William, Fort Bragg. On October 7, 1995, he killed one soldier and wounded 18 others. (Trib. Review, Sept.8, 2022) [He] had become hostile recently and had been previously seen by a military psychiatrist. According to the Washington Post (05.31, 1996) he "became depressed in 1994" and "received counselling for six months." He was a national honor student. A teacher described him as "a wonderful, young, top student" (Washington Post, cited in the Tribune Review, October 29, 1995) The victim's wife stated: "What drives a man to do that...I don't know. I can only have compassion for him and hope he gets the help he needs."

Lanza, Adam, 20, Newton, CT. He killed his mother, 20 children and 6 more adults in Sandy Hook and committed suicide. According to the Washington Post, (no date avail.) he was on medication as a neighbor recalled. He had been diagnosed with Asperger's syndrome when he was 13, anxiety in middle school and with

OCD when he was 14. He was prescribed <u>Celexa</u> but later stopped taking it. (Wikipedia)

<u>Lopez, Ivan</u>, Fort Hood, Texas, killed three, injured sixteen. He had sought help for depression and anxiety. (Associated Press, Trib. Review, no date avail.) "He was … undergoing regular psychiatric treatments for depression, anxiety and PTSD"(Wikipedia)

<u>Lubitz, Andreas</u>, the German pilot who locked himself into the cockpit and caused the death of all passengers and the crew. According to CNN they found <u>antidepressants</u> in his apartment. (March 28, 2015) and he had been hospitalized for depression (according to Wikipedia.)

<u>The Meidinger- Dougherty</u> case in 2010 in Greensburg, PA. ("The Greensburg six.") At least some of the defendants had mental health problems. According to Wikipedia and other sources:

> "<u>Melvin Knight</u> developed lifelong learning and social problems after he fell out of a moving vehicle and hit his head at age 5."

> The Tribune Review cited a psychologist (Nov.14, 2018) in regard to Knight: "he was diagnosed with depression, psychosis, substance abuse, attention deficit disorder and antisocial behavior." His mother stated: "He was first diagnosed at age 6". (Pittsburgh Post Gazette, Dec.4, 2020

> <u>Angela Marinucci</u> injured her head at age 15. Two mental health expert testified that as a child she suffered from depression.

> <u>Amber Meidinger</u>. Dr. Laura Labay, a toxicologist in their trial, testified "that Daugherty might have ingested up to 47 <u>Zoloft</u> pills - an antidepressant- in the hour before her death." "Police found Meidinger's empty Zoloft pill bottle during a search of the apartment. Labay said there were also traces of an antipsychotic, <u>Seroquel,</u> in Daugherty's system…A pharmacist at the Giant Eagle at Eastgate Plaza in Hempfield, Greensburg, PA, testified that Marinucci picked up a Seroquel prescription a month before the slaying" (Trib. Review, April 25, 2012)

> <u>Ricky Smyrnes</u> : "He was treated for mental health disorders as early as age 4. [He] had been diagnosed with PTSD (after sexual abuse) and had

undergone 103 therapy sessions by the age of 10…He was diagnosed with…seven different personalities and 15 total psychiatric issues." (Wikipedia, last edited, April 13, 2024)

O'Connor, Zachary, 25, died by suicide. He had been diagnosed with Attention Deficit Disorder (Trib. Review, Sept. 8, 2022)

Plaskon, Christopher, 17, in Milford, CT, stabbed a classmate to death. His lawyer: "He is on a laundry list of medication" (youtube.com "Prom day suspect pleads not guilty", June 4, 2014)

Qi, Tailei, was a student who shot his chemistry professor. According to "The Week "(Sept. 8, 2023) he had struggled with mental illness.

Redner, George, paramedic in Levittown near Philadelphia, committed suicide. His mother said: "He had been treated for mental health issues before" (Tribune Review, March19, 2017)

Remaley, Jacob, from New Stanton, PA , 14 at the time of the murder (in 2016), killed his mother and brother. He received a sentence of 30 years to life. "Remaley was diagnosed with multiple personality disorder and, according to his doctor, was under the influence of one." (Trib. Review, Feb. 25, 2020)

Routh, Ray killed "American sniper" author Chris Kyle and his friend, Chad Littlefield. Before the killing happened, "The VA first diagnosed him as having PTSD, according to his medical records. Doctors prescribed him Risperidone, an antipsychotic, as well as other medications to treat depression…He also stopped taking his medication, saying that the drugs made him feel like a "f……g zombie." (Newsweek Magazine, Nov. 23, 2015)

Sabbatino, Joseph, committed suicide. His father told KABC-TV that he had struggled with depression and had been prescribed medication." (Tribune Review, 3.19.16)

Schlemmer, Laurel, McCandless, PA., a former teacher. She drowned two sons in April 2014. She had been diagnosed with major depression disorder. (KDKA, March 16, 2017)

Sebek, Frank, 25, posted nude pictures of a former girlfriend on the Internet. He told the judge that "he has suffered with mental illness since he was 10…. and throughout his childhood and into adulthood and diagnosed with attention deficit disorder, depression and severe anxiety disorder." (He had also made several suicide attempt.) (Trib. Review, April 29, 1922)

Seung Hui Cho, killed 32 people, died by suicide. He had been in psychiatric hospital and was ordered to receive treatment. "in middle school he was diagnosed with severe anxiety disorder with selective mutism (DSM definition of selective mutism: "Failure to speak when there is an expectation to speak (in school) if persons speak in other situations".(This diagnosis does not take the possible cultural background into account) as well as manic depressive disorder. After his diagnosis he began to receive treatment. His parents sought treatment for him through medication and therapy." (Wikipedia)

Shell, Shawn: he was a psychiatric patient at Mayview hospital and died of a heatstroke. Dr. Carl Werner stated "Drugs commonly given to mental patients, including some anti – depressants, are known to contribute to heat stroke." (Trib. Review, Aug. 18, 1995)

Thompson, Nigel, 14 at the time of the murder in 2023 (he killed another boy). "By the time he was 13, Nigel Thompson has been hospitalized twice at UPMC-Western Psychiatric Hospital."(Trib. Live , April4 4, 2024.

Treacy, Wayne, Fort Lauderdale : On Oct. 23, 2012 ,when he was 15, he kicked and stomped a fifteen- year-old in the head. (over an argument or taunting about his brother's suicide that had happened not long before). He had been an honor student, but after his brother's death he suffered post traumatic stress, depression and suicidal thoughts." (source not avail.) Was he treated for this? Psychologist Michael Brannon said: "Treacy should have been on medication to treat previously diagnosed attention-deficit hyperactivity disorder." (The Palm Beach Post, April 1, 2012). "He cried during the trial" (Sun Sentinel, June 16, 2018). The judge ordered medication for PTSD.

Uyesugi, Brian, 40, Honolulu, shot seven members of his work team. He had undergone psychiatric treatment according to the No. 2, 99 Hawaiian News.: "We are looking into reports that Uyesugi had undergone psychiatric treatment."

Wesbecker, Joseph Thomas, Louisville, Kentucky (s. Glenmillen, chapter 20) : He killed eight people and wounded twelve before committing suicide. "In August

1989, less than a month before the shooting, Wesbecker had started to take Prozac. The wounded and the families of those killed filed a law suit against manufacturer Ely Lilly and company, claiming that Wesbecker's use of Prozac had contributed to his actions. (Wikipedia. org cited in Murderpedia.org) Psychiatrist Joseph Glenmullen commented: "But new information has come to light that the pharmaceutical giant has paid millions of dollars to victims and survivors of Prozac-related suicides and murders. One victim received a huge amount of money that was only revealed in his divorce proceeding. "(Glenmullen, chapter 20.) The jury decided 9:3 for Lilly.

These are just random cases, there are many more.

In all of these cases psychotropic drugs or psychological treatment are involved. As we can see they even endanger public figures like President Reagan. (I could not find any information on the shootings of representative Gabby Giffords on January 8, 2011 that resulted in the death of six people and injuries of 13.) About the recent attempt on President Trump's life, TRIBLIVE wrote about the shooter, Thomas Matthew Crooks, : "He also searched for information about major depression disorder, the sources told news outlets." (TRIBLIVE, July19,2024))

The public should know that the treatment usually only means a prescription rather than a discussion with a psychiatrist. It is much cheaper to do that. My heart goes out to people who have lost children to suicide or violent attacks, but also to the parents or relatives of people who have committed these violent acts under the influence of psychotropic drugs. The public should be informed that medication for mental problems have only been tested for a short time, that the FDA warns of the side effects, including unusual behavior and aggression and that huge profits are gained by what I call the mental health industry. Our children involved are the victims. They are prescribed medications, are not being warned (although the FDA recommends or even requires it) and they do not know why they are doing what they are doing. Many of them spend the rest of their life in confinement. How come America has more school shootings than any other country? (How come other countries forbid, e.g. drugs like "Adderall"?)

Let me cite the Ground Report in this regard:

The Ground Report, a digital News platform, stated on Nov. 16, 2022

> "Since 1970 when current records began, there have been 2155 school shootings in the United States that left 661 dead. Last year figures reached an all- time high with more than 250 incidents recorded, an increase of 120% from the previous year when 114 incidents were reported. 2022 is already the worst year on record. More than 600 mass shootings this year." (2022)

And in regard to suicides, there were more than 50 000 in 2023, more than in any previous year. (Meet the press, NBC,12.31.2023)

Taking a closer look at the previous cases, one observation becomes clear: Many of the adolescents who committed the killings came from terrible homes or experienced great sadness in their lives. The recent death of his parents in Nikolas Cruz' case, the court ordered use of Luvox in Eric Harris' and Dylan Klebold's case, a brother's suicide in Wayne Treacy's case or the prescribing of psychotropical drugs to members of the Greensburg six. These are examples were adolescents were found guilty and have to spend years in prison or even will receive the death penalty. Even more tragic are the murders committed by children, sometimes as young as eleven (Jordan Brown.) According to the Dept. of Justice:

> "In 2020 there were 930 people 17 and younger arrested on murder charges." (Trib. Review, August 3, 2024)

These children are treated as adults
They have been prescribed these medications, they did not take them voluntarily (sometimes under codes that are not even valid, like poverty. (See DSM codes V and Z). The really guilty are the prescribers and the legal authorities who are misinformed about the side effects although these are listed and easily accessible. The guilty are the pharmaceutical companies who often hide or falsify the side effects, the FDA who allows off label use and the politicians who accept great contributions from the corporations. Not many, except a few courageous people, like psychiatrist Peter Breggin, stand up for these children or adolescents.
We often neglect these young people when they grow up in terrible homes and we abandon them when they have been caught in the very dangerous net of these psychiatric drugs.

What should be done:

1. Each case should be examined as to what medication was used.
2. The public should be informed of this and the side effects.
3. "Unusual behavior" and "aggression" should be examined more closely.
4. Other approaches, like talk therapy, should be taken to help troubled youth.

In the following I want to examine the pathway that led to the creation of the DSM, the book on which the identification and treatment of mental illness is largely based.

3. Emil Kraepelin, his influence on modern psychiatry and criticism of his work

The DSM, the manual that is used to identify mental disorders, that I will discuss in one of the following chapters, is based to a great extent on Emil Kraepelin. He is often called "the father of psychiatry."

Emil Kraepelin (1856 - 1926) was born in the State of Mecklenburg, Germany. According to Wikipedia, he is considered to be the founder of modern scientific psychiatry and psychopharmacology and psychiatric genetics. He developed "a large scale, clinically oriented epidemiological research programme." (Wikipedia accessed on 3.29. 2023.) His major work "Ein Lehrbuch der Psychiatrie" was first published in 1883. It was followed by numerous multi volumes of new editions. "He started to establish the <u>foundations of the modern classification system</u>. He felt that by studying case histories and identifying special disorders, the progression of mental disorders could be predicted. His final edition comprised four volumes and was published in 1927." (Wikipedia, accessed on Jan. 5, 2024)

The psychiatrist James <u>Walter Dennert</u> writes about Kraepelin "Despite the problems scholars have pointed out with Kraepelin's work, many of his clinical findings form the basis for modern understanding of mental illnesses...the main features of his classification system continues to exist in many current international classification systems of mental disorders, such as the Diagnostic and Statistical Manual of Mental Disorders-5 (DSM-5) and the International Classification of Diseases 10.(ICD - 10) ." (Dennert, Walter James "Emil Kraepelin (1856-1926), Embryo Project Encyclopedia, publ. 2021-05-07")

Before I submit my own examination of Kraepelin's classification system I want to cite other authors who are critical of his classification of mental disorders, mostly psychiatrist <u>Stephan Heckers</u> from Vanderbilt University who cites other psychiatrists. He writes about Kraepelin: (Source not found)

- He "published a thoughtful critique of his own classification system."

- He <u>created</u> diseases (<u>Adolf Meyer</u>). In his 8th edition his "dementia praecox " had grown from three to eleven subtypes and the book from 107 to 354 pages. (Heckers)
- In his classification Kraepelin neglected the "whole person and his or her life story."(Kender et al)
- He often blamed missing willpower in his patients (Dennert)
- His patient reports were already interpretations of a disease. (Weber and Engstrom, cited in Heckers.) In other words, Kraepelin did not observe behaviors first before making a decision about a disease.
- Already during Kraepelin's lifetime some supposedly mental disorders were identified as having biological causes like Syphillis. (Heckers)
- "Cerebral processes with somatic manifestations had always been identified on the basis of physical examinations rather than psychopathological theorizing... Any assessment of all the clinical evidence could not culminate in clearly defined diseases ... it would produce only different types of disorders ...that were characterized by transitional or borderline symptoms."(Kender) He disputes Kraepelin's claim that common outcomes could serve as evidence of common diseases. Kender points out that a connection between molecular processes and reactions of the human body are not understood. He concludes that Kraepelin's system "continues to shape our field... fruitful for the young science of psychiatry, but...their ultimate value remains to be determined." (Kenneth Kender, MD, Eric Engstrom, PHD "Criticism of Kraepelin's Psychiatric Nosology: 1896-1927" in The American Journal of Psychiatry, published online October 15, 2017.)
- <u>Hannah Decker</u>, professor of history, quotes Kraepelin himself : "There are no fixed but only blurred borders between mental health and mental illness."(in "How Kraepelinian was Kraepelin? How Kraepelinian are the neo-Kraepelinians?-from Emil Kraepelin to DSM-III, History of Psychiatry 2007, 18, p.341)
- "But for the majority of psychiatric disorders biological validation was not available to Kraepelin and <u>is still lacking today</u>" (Heckers)
- Psychiatric clinicians and researchers often assess validation differently (Heckers)

4. My examination of Kraepelin's classification system and his treatments

For my examination of Kraepelin's classification system I used the edition listed in the bibliography.

(I left out the following diseases that he described : epilepsy, alcoholism, morphinism, and cocainism, insanity in acute diseases like from brain lesions or head injuries, senility, criminality, imbecility and cretinism, because some of these are clearly organic , some are addiction issues and some have causes that have not been solved.)

I was taken aback when I read how Kraepelin had treated his patients. They were introduced in a lecture hall to his students. He described them and their peculiarities in their presence and often also their relatives, in unflattering terms. He pricked them with a needle, sometimes into their eye-lids (p. 132) or he poured water on them (p. 83). He often used artificial feeding. He can't understand why the patients sometimes react violently or are apprehensive (after all, most of them were locked up against their will) and he lists these reactions as signs of a mental disease.

In my opinion Kraepelin does not act in a scientific way. Most of the time is spent with anecdotes about what the patient did and descriptions of his/her relatives who, he claims, were also insane, without checking the individual cases. From there, he deduces that mental illness is inherited, a claim that has, unfortunately, influenced the thinking of some relatives of mental patients and professionals and has not been validated. He names the previous hospital and asylum confinements and lists the treatment he used. It does not seem to occur to him that the treatment they received previously or under his care probably caused the very symptoms of the disease he describes. (I will look at these in detail). And finally, there is a danger of inadequate translation from the German into English, e.g. what do you do with a sentence part like this :" … departure from the average in the direction of efficiency…" (p.295) [Although the meaning can be guessed when you continue reading. (p. 295 ff.)

In the chapters that I examined I found 47 cases of mental illness. Of those, 27 persons had spent time in a hospital or asylum and had been treated with medication, sometimes prolonged bathing or salt infusions. Some had previously suffered from syphilis or typhus and were therefore treated with mercury or Atoxyl.

Here is a list of treatments and medications that Kraepelin applied and their side effect (I used the literature in the NIH (National Institute for Health) in most cases, in other cases Wikipedia and other sources):

<u>Drug</u>:   <u>Side effect</u>:

<u>Atoxyl</u>   Is an arsenic compound, can cause blindness, head tremors, incoordination, euphoria, ataxia (loss of coordination), paraparesis, (loss of voluntary motion) etc. (Paul E. Miller "Food Animal practice, 5th ed., 2009)

<u>Alcohol</u>   Can affect the way the brain works

<u>Bromide of Sodium (NaBr)</u>   Can cause, among others, drowsiness, irritability, incoordination, vertigo, confusion, mania, slurred speech, hallucinations, tremor, psychosis. (website Santa Cruz Biotechnology) "…as a hypnotic, anticonvulsant and sedative widely used in medicine in the late 19th and 20th century" (Wikipedia) Kraepelin : [We have given] "the patient 12 and then 15 grammes of bromide of sodium daily on the first symptom of excitement… doses of hyoscine or sulphonal are often necessary…"(p.67) But later on he warns "The danger of bromide poisoning must not be overlooked. To consume large quantities of bromides without a doctor's prescription … is a very dangerous measure." (p.245)

Camphor   Can induce seizures (NIH)

Cocaine   Paranoid delusions, illusions of insects crawling...
                               (Wikipedia)

Hyoscine   made from Belladonna alkaloid. Can cause
                               psychosis (NIH). "Child experienced
                               hallucinations" was agitated and restless "the
                               cognitive deficiencies were remarkable" (Clinical
                               case report PMID 35540718 –publ. online in May
                               2022)

Hypnotics   Sedatives, can cause unusual behavior, cognitive
                               dysfunction (Wikipedia)

Iodide of potassium   or Iodine, can cause shrinkage of thyroid gland
                               and decrease in the amount of thyroid
                               hormones (WebMD) "...which at any rate is
                               harmless"(Kraepelin, p.44)

Mercury   Neurotoxin symptoms (among others):
                               impairment of speech and/or walking, tremors,
                               emotional changes like excessive shyness,
                               twitching, poor performance in tests, mental
                               disturbances. "Can cause neurological damage
                               that leads to hallucinations and psychosis"
                               (Medicalnewstoday.com/articles/320563#outlook)

Mercurial inunction   Treatment with mercury fumes, (Kraepelin,
                               p.366) "now considered to be so toxic, that gas
                               masks have to be worn when dealing with
                               them." (Richter, p.18)

Opium   Sedation and decreased cognition (NIH)

Paraldehyde   "Can produce narcotic effect with some diminution of consciousness" (NIH)

Sulphonal   Hypnotic drug, causes mood or mental changes (Mayo clinic) Can cause giddiness, staggering gait, paralysis (Wikipedia)

Trional   is a sedative, hypnotic, can cause unconsciousness, i.e. inability to maintain awareness of self and environment (Wikipedia)

Kraepelin writes about one of his mental patients, describing this patient's statements: "He had to take great quantities of quicksilver (Mercury) and that poisoned him" (p.47) "Poison was put into his food to stupefy him and make him crazy" (p.47) Kraepelin mocks this man and thinks that his statements are a sign of the man's insanity. Nowadays science would agree with the patient.

5. My criticism of Kraepelin

- He mostly uses cases of patients who had been treated before with medication that causes mental disturbances to say the least, or were treated with these medications for syphilis or typhus. Often, they have spent months or years in an asylum and have been treated with mercury or highly toxic substances.
- He claims that mental diseases are inherited without researching the cases of the relatives (they probably have been treated with mind altering drugs just like the cases before him)
- Already here it can be seen that there is no clear distinction between the mental diseases, like:
    Delirium
    Delusion
    Dementia
    Depression (apprehensive, circular, manic)
    Hallucinations
    Hysteria
    Katatonia
    Mania, manical depressive insanity, manical excitement, manical depressive
        excitement
    Megalomania
    Melancholia
    Paralysis
    Paranoia

- Kraepelin writes that some diseases are due to an impediment of thought and will. (like in circular depression)
- His diagnostics are not clearly defined which can cause misdiagnosis and dangerous treatment. This leads to confusion among diagnosticians. In tests it has been shown that often there was no agreement among diagnosticians to identify a mental disease. (s. lately the Bower's case, chapter 2.)
- In his defense I want to quote Kraepelin :" In such "stationary" [paralysis] cases emphasis must always be laid on the probability of mistakes in the diagnosis,

especially in the confusion of general paralysis with syphilitic lesions of the cortex"(p. 199) and

"a single symptom, however characteristic it may be, never justifies a definite diagnosis by itself,...only the whole picture can ever be decisive of the clinical hypothesis" (p.278) (my emphasis) and

"The standard we use in recognising the morbid features of a man's mental life is his departure from the average in the direction of inefficiency" (p. 295)

What should be done in regard to the DSM characterization of symptoms:

1. All cases that have been treated with medication that can cause mental diseases should be disregarded
2. A new system of classification should be created that only lists and categorizes symptoms that appear in untreated cases
3. This classification system should be conducted by experts who are totally independent from outside influences, namely from corporations, politicians etc.

6. The DSM-5, the ICD-10 and my criticism

The authoritative guide for identifying mental disorders are the (current) DSM-5 TR (Diagnostic and Statistical Manual of Mental Disorders, Text Revision) and the ICD-10 (International Classification of Diseases). As stated, the DSM is used for identifying mental disorders, whereas the ICD-10 is used to provide the codes for billing purposes. The DSM -5 TR has been published on March 18, 2022, (the DSM -5 had been published on May 18, 2013) It follows previous editions. It contains close to 300 mental disorders and is used by psychiatrists, mental health professionals, the judicial system and health insurances. Each of the listed disorders has a code which is used for treatment recommendations, insurance reimbursements and also in legal proceedings. For instance, it can be used to deny somebody a job, commit persons or to decide in child custody cases or take children from parents who were labelled mentally disordered. In other words, it can greatly influence or even change a person's life.

The DSM is based, as mentioned, to a great extent on a classification system created by Emil Kraepelin about 100 years ago. Kraepelin observed mental patients, wrote down their symptoms and created his list. When you read some of his classifications, you might already see that they were influenced by the popular thinking of his time. For instance, not wanting to serve in the army was considered a mental disease. (Is it really healthier to have no qualms about killing somebody or to witness terrible suffering and blood spilling?) Kraepelin wrote eight editions of his textbook and doubted some classifications himself later as we saw.

The previous DSM III, followed by the DSM IV, used a multi-axial system which included physical disorders (axis III), psychosocial stresses (axis IV) and level of functioning (axis V).

Robert Spitzer, the originator of the DSM III added 25 diagnostic criteria. They were meant to be suggestive, not binding, and were supposed to add "diagnostic reliability." The result was that the diagnostic reliability was only deemed acceptable for 3 items: Mental deficiency, organic brain syndrome and alcoholism and fair for psychosis and schizophrenia. For every other category it was extremely poor" (Decker, p.352)

"Objections were raised from several sources. DSM III was said to be anti-humanistic, failing to do justice to the complexity of the human mind" (Decker, p. 353)

Today, the DSM-5 is used together with the ICD-10 which is used in all WHO countries for mental disorders. (The code CM that sometimes follows the ICD-10 means "clinically modified." All ICD-10 and ICD-10-CM are appropriated for billing but not for diagnosing mental health disorders)

I am going to name the different health codes that are listed in the ICD-10-CM (which, as pointed out, are used by the health insurances). I am doing this because I want you to be able to determine if some categories that are listed under Mental Disorders (F- code) really belong there.

A and B   = infections and parasitic diseases (ds)

C and D   =neoplasms (abnormal growth of tissue, like cancer)

E   =endocrine, nutritional, metabolic diseases

F   **=mental and behavioral disorders**

G   =nervous system ds. (most sleep and wake ds.)

H   =eye and ear ds.

I   =circulatory system ds.

J   =respiratory system ds.

K   =digestive system ds.

L   =skin ds.

M   =musculoskeletal ds.

N   =genitourinary ds.

O   =pregnancy, childbirth and puerperium ds.

P   =in the perinatal period

Q   =congenital malformation

R   =symptoms and...abnormal lab findings

S and T   =injury etc. as consequences of external causes, physical abuse

V, W, X, Y   =external causes of morbidity

> <u>V-code</u> is not a diagnosis but a supplementary classification of factors influencing health status and contact with health services circumstances other than the disease. "Might have negative impact on mental health"

Z   =factors influencing health status and contact with health services similar to current V-codes.) Used for circumstances other than disease, injury or external use. (Might be used for vaccination, e.g.)

    <u>PsychDB</u> (Psychiatry Data Base), (https://:psychdb.com) (* s. back of book) remarks "that V and Z codes <u>are not mental disorders</u> … there is often a lack of awareness about these codes. It is often helpful to put V and Z codes in a patient's clinical documentation when there is no evidence of a mental disorder, but if they are presenting with significant impairment."

    So the Z codes, e.g. Z 596 (low income) problems (or Z 55 (related to education and literacy) <u>do not indicate a disorder</u> but are often treated as one, in other words, children or adolescents could be treated with dangerous psychiatric drugs when unwarranted.

(Question: What is the difference between F (mental and behavioral disorders) and G (nervous system disorders?)

    As mentioned, the DSM lists about 300 diseases and contains groups and subgroups of disorders.

There are 21 groups of mental disorders:

<u>Neurodevelopmental Disorders</u> (like stuttering)

<u>Schizophrenic Spectrum and Other Psychotic Disorders</u> (like Delusional Disorder)

<u>Bipolar and Related Disorders</u>

<u>Depressive Disorders</u> (like Premenstrual Dysphoric Disorder)

<u>Anxiety Disorders</u> (like Selective Mutism)

27

Obsessive-Compulsive and Related Disorders (like Hoarding Disorder)

Trauma and Stressor Related Disorder (like Adjustment Disorder)

Dissociative Disorders

Somatic Symptoms and Related Disorders (like Illness Anxiety Disorder)

Feeding and Eating Disorders (like Bulimia)

Elimination Disorders

Sleep – Wake Disorder: (like insomnia)

Sexual Dysfunctions (like Female Orgasmic Disorder)

Gender Dysphoria

Disruptive, Impulse-Control and Conduct Disorders (like Kleptomania)

Substance Related and Addictive Disorders (like Caffeine Intoxication)

Neurocognitive Disorders (like: Due to Alzheimer Disease)

Personality Disorders (like Narcissistic Personality Disorder)

Paraphilic Disorder (like Exhibitionistic Disorder)

Other Mental Disorders

Medication – induced Movement Disorder and Other Adverse Effect of Medication

As I mentioned previously, psychiatric professionals and the public seem to be confused about the terms used in psychiatry. I used the definitions in DSM-5 to examine some of these terms:

ADHD:	Persistent pattern of inattention and/or hyperactivity – impulsivity that interferes with functioning or development

Anxiety	Excessive worry and apprehensive expectation, occurring more days than not for at least 6 months about a number of events or activities such as work or school performance

Bipolar	Group of brain disorders that cause extreme fluctuations in a person's mood, energy and ability to function
Delirium	A disturbance of attention, i.e. reduced ability to direct, focus, sustain and shift attention and awareness and reduced attention to environment
Delusion	Fixed beliefs that are not amenable to change in light of conflicting evidence
Depression	Feeling of sadness or low mood and loss of interest in their usual activities. Must mark a change from a person's previous level of functioning and have persisted for at least 2 weeks.
Hallucination	Defined as a sensory perception in the absence of a corresponding external or somatic stimulus and described according to the sensory domain in which it occurs
Mania	Distinct period of abnormally and persistently increased goal – directed activity or energy
Paranoia	Individuals who have a pervasive, persistent and enduring mistrust of others and profoundly cynical view of others and the world
Psychosis	Presence of one (or more) of the following symptoms: delusions, hallucinations, disorganized speech (e.g. frequent derailment or incoherence, grossly disorganized or catatonic behavior)
Schizophrenia	A chronic mental illness with positive symptoms (delusions, hallucinations, disorganized speech and behavior, negative symptoms and cognitive impairment)

Each sub segment includes a "unspecified "section, e.g. "unspecified intellectual disability" that leaves the reader at a loss about the meaning,

If you take a closer look at these categories, you will notice that

1.) some are hardly discernable from others, e.g. under ADHD "inattention" and under Delirium "disturbance of attention"

2.) some claim scientific explanations that are <u>not proven</u>, e.g. under "Bipolar: group of brain disorders"

3.) nebulous, e.g. under Hallucination "and described according to the sensory domain in which it occurs" or under Anxiety "more days than not for at least 6 months" or "excessive worry and apprehensive expectation". (how much worry is just right?)

The danger here is a misdiagnosis by an expert, a mistaken belief of a patient in the veracity of the carelessly used scientific claims and a missing understanding by a patient of nebulous terms.

The manual does not suggest certain medications for specific disorders and it is being admitted <u>that medication does not heal the disorder but only deals with the symptoms,</u> as stated in <u>WebMd</u>, a government publication. It seems to me that the symptoms can be healed, but not the disorder because we don't know where the disorder originates. There are about 100 billion of brain cells (according to the NIH) about which we know very little. And we cannot even be sure that the symptoms are cured. Does somebody with agoraphobia suddenly like to go out in the public? Does a person with ADHD suddenly become more successful? Have any studies been conducted to prove these assumptions?

So disorders like depression and anxiety cannot be healed, but only their symptoms can be treated, mostly with SSRI medication, a medication that will be discussed later.

I have taken a closer look at some of the sub - disorders listed in the DSM-5. I have used their definitions or parts of them for which I used quotation marks and added my comment in parenthesis.

As you will see many disorders are common human reactions to events that cause stress, the "fight or flight" or Freud's pain/pleasure principle, the reactions that make us human. The danger is that many will interpret these in themselves and their children as anomalies and subject themselves to dangerous and mind damaging treatment.

- Adjustment Disorder: "…Emotional or behavioral symptoms in response to an identifiable stressor" There is medication to lessen symptoms: Benzodiazepines like Ativan or Xanax and non benzodiazepines like Neurontin. (This is much too general and can be widely interpreted. Is a stressor always identifiable and is there not always a reaction to a stressor? - the definition of stress is that it causes stress.)

- Anxiety: "Excessive worry…"(Again, how much worry is acceptable?)

- Avoidant Personality Disorder: "Avoidance of any involvement with other people unless certain they will be liked"
 (Don't we all have a tendency to do this? "I love to go out with her: she hates me and always criticizes me! "(Freud's pleasure/pain principle!)

- Body Dysmorphic Disorder "Preoccupation with… perceived defects or flaws in physical appearance" (To some extent we all do that but especially teenagers!)

- Caffeine Intoxication: "Health professionals recommend daily intake "restricted] to …just over 4 cups of …coffee." Use of beta blockers is recommended. (Many people drink that much coffee-a mental disorder?)

- Conduct Disorder "behavior where the rights of others or…societal…rules…are violated" (what is the difference to "Oppositional Defiant Disorder"?) (Rights of other are constantly violated —like in wars - that is unfortunately human nature.)

- Conversion Disorder: "Altered motor functions" (could be side effects of psychotropic medication, like tics or Tourette syndrome.)

- Cyclothymic "periods of elevated mood and depressive symptoms for at least 2 years. The symptoms occur at least half the time" – there is no medication for this approved by the FDA, but doctor may prescribe medication for bipolar disorder. (The symptoms sound like bipolar disorder to me, use of difficult terms like "cyclothymic" that might keep professional from looking word up and therefore make a faulty diagnosis)

- Dependent Personality Disorder: "excessive need to be taken care of, submissive…" (What is "excessive"? Who makes that judgment? Don't we all want to be taken care of, receive love and acceptance?)

- Depersonalization: "Detachment with respect to one's thoughts etc." (What do they mean by that?)

- Disinhibited Social Engagement "Reduced or absent reticence in approaching and interacting with unfamiliar adults" No medication, but possible connection to ADHD for which, (of course) there is medication. (What is just the correct distance one should keep in social engagement, because there is also Selective Mutism – the hesitancy of a child to talk to relatives that the child hasn't seen for a long time)

- Disruptive Mood Dysregulation (under depression) "severe recurrent temper outbursts", the antidepressant Celexa is recommended. (Why is this listed under depression? Almost every parent had to deal with these-remember the "terrible two"? Danger of parents to treat child with this very dangerous drug just to make things easier.)

- Female Sexual Interest Arousal Disorder (could have physical reasons or temporary psychological reasons (like too tired, too old, mad at somebody)) Treating it with a psychotic drug could avoid patient seeking treatment for an organic cause or figure out a solution to a problem.

- Gender Dysphobia: "Distress or impairment related to gender incongruence (not all transgender or gender diverse experience…[this]" (May be a person has to sort their feelings out on this and doing this is not a mental disease.)

- Genito-Pelvic Pain Disorder: (Should first be checked for organic causes.)

- Global Development Delay – "when an individual fails to meet expected developmental milestones in several areas of intellectual functioning" (is there a test for each milestone and for each area?)

- Illness Anxiety: "preoccupation with the idea that one has or will get a serious illness with lack of somatic illness" "…If the patient is in a high risk category for e.g. heart disease but there are no current indicators of heart disease … the patient's anxiety is out of proportion." "SSRIs may be useful" (Theravive) (Flies into face of reason: Cancer, diabetes etc. show connection to genes- and health professionals often ask if these diseases "have been in the family." To ignore that is downright dangerous.)

- Insomnia (Could be symptoms of so many other organic disease, e.g. cancer and should be carefully examined.)

- Major or Mild Neurocognitive Disorder due to traumatic brain injury. (This is a clearly somatic disease]

- Major Depressive Disorder "Depressed mood, loss of interest and pleasure, agitation." (A loaded definition, will be discussed later)

- Nightmare (could be side effect of several psychotropic medications, e.g. for tobacco cessation)

- Obstructive Sleep Apnea (Again, clearly a somatic disease)

- Oppositional Defiant Disorder: "angry, irritable mood, argumentative, defiant behavior…high comorbidity with ADHD" (therefor can be treated with psychotroic drugs – (again, a disregard of possible stages a youth goes through and actually should go through to mature)

- Paranoia: "Individuals who have a pervasive, persistent and enduring mistrust of others and profoundly cynical view of others and the world." (Tries to impose a world view that is positive and uncritical. Totally ignores religions

(Buddhism, Christianity) and philosophers. Did Teddy Roosevelt's "Carry a big stick" or Rome's "Lupus homini lupus est" (Wolf is wolf to man) show paranoia?

- <u>Premenstrual Dysphonic Disorder</u> (This is clearly a purely physical affliction due to hormonal influence and should not be listed here)

- <u>Reactive Attachment Disorder</u> "chronic pattern of being emotionally withdrawn...demonstrated by rarely seeking or responsive to comfort when distressed" (this could be the case with a child in a dysfunctional family or abusive foster care or even could be a cultural issue and should be investigated and treated with care and love, not with psychiatric drugs.)

- <u>Restless Leg Syndrome:</u> (clearly a somatic disease, could be lack of calcium-so much research has to be done in regard to muscles.)

- <u>Schizo Affective</u> (under debate, sounds like schizophrenia with a good <u>outcome), schizophreniform</u> "at least one of delusion, hallucination, disorganized speech for a significant time during a one month period" <u>and</u> <u>schizophrenia</u> "at least two of delusion, hallucination, disorganized speech." (Too many subgroups, how long is "significant time"?)

- <u>Selective Mutism</u> "Failure to speak when there is an expectation to speak (in school) if persons speaks in other situations. (There can be so many reasons, e.g. not being sure of the answer, not to appear to be a teacher's pet in front of other students etc.)

- <u>Separation anxiety</u> "Persistent reluctance to go out." (Difference to agoraphobia?)

- <u>Social Anxiety for (most of the day)</u> "fear... about social situation, because of fear to be judged negatively" (Totally normal behavior - don't we all have this fear? s. Freud's pleasure/pain principle.)

- Social Communication Disorder "deficits such as greeting and information …appropriate for social context "(fails to take different cultural and family values into account. What is social context? Is it really safe to talk to strangers?)

- Stimulant Use Disorder: "the continuous use of amphetamine- type …leading to …impairment or distress." (This listing is ironic because so many people (and children!) are prescribed amphetamines like Aderall or Ritalin!]

- Stuttering
  (as far as I know it is a physical disease, not a mental one. There was an English king and an American president who had this affliction]

- Tobacco Use
  (A mental disease?)

What is common to almost all of these disorders:

1. Missing scientific proof (no chemical or missing chemical found in body)
2. Nebulous, unscientific, illogical, circular language is used to describe the disorder
3. Scientific sounding expressions using latinized or greek terms (like cyclothymic) that can confuse laymen and even experts. These can give them seeming authority.

The danger is, that patient will not seek medical answer or are rarely given the opportunity for "Talk therapy" (because of insurance cost).

7. What does the ideal (mentally healthy) person look like according to the DSM?

I have constructed such a person who is mentally healthy in the eyes of the DSM :

- Does not have somatic diseases like restless leg syndrome, genito-pelvic pain, insomnia, night mares, sleep apnea, premenstrual pain, does not stutter.

- Does not care if people don't like him/her.

- Doesn't care what he/she looks like.

- Does not want to be taken care of.

- His/her mind never wanders- he/she always concentrates on just one thing.

- He/she always finds the correct distance to people-not too close, not too distant.

- Never gets depressed, anxious or sad. (like Lincoln)

- Does not get nervous before public speaking. (the no.1 fear in general.)

- Is not sad longer than a certain time when a loved one dies.

- Is not afraid of diseases, even when at high risk because of genes, if there is no current indicator of the disease.

- Always is ready to have sex.

- Does not indulge in coffee, alcohol, food, the Internet. (Remember, there are limits, like 4 cups of coffee.)

- Always pays attention, even if speaker or teacher is boring. (not like Tom Sawyer or Huckleberry Finn.)

- Is not influenced by his culture. (Some cultures discourage to be too outgoing!)

- Does not become sad because of events like death, poverty, crime, injustice.

(I am convinced that the experts soon will come up with the mental disorder label "Too normal"!)

You end up with a Mr. Goody-two shoes, a person without a heart or a soul. (I call this a marble statue model.) Do you want to have a friend like this or do you want to be that person?

How many heroes or heroines in literature would be labelled mentally disordered if they would be measured by DSM standards (Hamlet, Natasha in "War and Peace" etc.,- so there would be very little literature left!) Should we consider them to be mentally disordered because they deal with and try to find a solution for human problems? Should we treat humans who are worried about those problems, and rob them of their humanity?

The sad part is that the perceived (by the DSM) faults can have serious legal consequences and terrible consequences for your health. Remember also, it is pointed out that the disorder cannot be healed, only the symptoms.

8. The people who created the DSM-5 according to the APA

That is the title that the American Psychiatric Association (APA), the group that is responsible for the writing, editing and publishing of the DSM, gives to an article on the Internet in 2013. (2013 AMA "The people behind the DSM-5"). In it, they claim that they

"began recruiting a roster of diverse and international-recognized clinicians, scientific researchers and organizations to lend their expertise… the DSM-5 development process has involved not only psychiatrists, but also experts with backgrounds in psychology, social work, psychiatric nursing, pediatrics and neurology." They represent 16 countries "All are leaders in their field and are participating on a voluntary basis." There is a task force of 28 and 13 work groups and more than 160 mental health and medicals "Each work group chair is a member of the task force…The work groups …have reviewed the scientific advances and research-based evidence that is the basis of the DMS…The work group members represent more than 90 academic and mental health institutions throughout the world." About 30% are international, 100 are psychiatrists, 47 psychologists, two are pediatric neurologists, three are statisticians /epidemiologists. There is a pediatrician, a speech and hearing specialist, a social worker, a psychiatric nurse and a consumer (?) and family representative.

There are more than <u>300 outside advisers</u> involved that have been requested by a work group "because of a specific and well recognized expertise in a particular field." They "are providing the task force and work groups with a wealth of knowledge based on their clinical and research experience."
There are two independent committees to review the DSM-5, a scientific Review Committee and a Clinical and Public Health committee. The draft of the DSM-5 has been "opened for public review "(there were nearly 11,000 comments) "Criteria have undergone rigorous testing at large academic medical centers."

When you read this description, you wonder who these "outside advisors" are. Are all the psychiatrists, psychologists and other expert not sufficient? They should be at the forefront of science. Could these "outside advisors" be paid by the drug companies and help to create diseases and medication for them? How else would we end up with exotic diseases like "social anxiety (for most of the day): fear… about social situation, because of fear to be judged negatively". We <u>all</u> have this fear. Or "bereavement disorder", which states that if you are sad longer than a few months after a loved one's death you have a mental disorder! Or premenstrual syndrome – clearly a matter of hormones! And remember – no disorder can be cured, only the symptoms. And every disorder has medication for it, mostly used off-label. Just check the following FDA-warnings! We cannot sit back and have theses dangerous medications often prescribed for "disorders" that are nothing else but normal human traits. Reading this article makes one wonder about all the people involved in the creation of the DSM. What does "organization", "all are leaders in their field" and especially "300 outside advisors" mean?

9. Financial conflict of interest in creating the DSM

(My article is based on the publication by <u>PLOS (Public Library of Science (plos.org))</u> which, according to Wikipedia, won't accept pharmaceutical advertisements or pharma-influenced articles, published online on March 13, 2012)

- The American Psychiatric Association (APA) instituted a financial conflict of interest disclosure policy for DSM-5.
- The policy has not been accompanied by a reduction in the financial conflicts of interest of the panel members
- There is a potential for bias, it does not protect the integrity of the revision process

Psychiatry is the epicenter of concerns of industry involvement like "ghostwriting" and failure to report industry-related income. "Some have wondered if the inclusion of new disorders, e.g. "Adjustment Disorder Related to Bereavement" reflects corporate interest."

The psychiatric disorders codified in the DSM have large public impact in regard to insurance, the law and the international classification of diseases.

While DSM-IV had no financial disclosure of their panel members, DSM-5 panel members are required to file financial disclosure statement which are expected to be listed in the publication. The APA has made a commitment to improve its management of financial conflicts of interest (FCOI) These data show a clear connection to funding sources whereby the results are favorably biased toward the interest of the funder. ("Funding effect"). This fact may encourage professionals and consumers to evaluate medical information more critically.

The DSM-5 task force was formed in 2007. In 2012, <u>69% of its members had ties</u> to the industry.

"Emerging data suggests that transparency of the funding source alone is an insufficient solution for eliminating bias."

<u>"3/4 of the work groups continue to have a majority of their members with ties to the pharmaceutical industry</u>. It is also

noteworthy that...the most conflicted panels are those for which pharmaceutical treatment is the first- line intervention. For example, 67% of the panel for mood disorders, 83 % of the panel for psychotic disorders and 100% of the sleep/wake disorders (which now includes "Restless Leg Syndrome") have ties to the pharmaceutical companies that manufacture the medications used to treat these disorders or to companies that service the pharmaceutical industry."

"When we did an internet search of 141 panel members we found that 15 %...were members of drug companies' speaker bureaus or advisory boards... Speaker bureau participation is usually prohibited elsewhere (e.g. for faculty in medical schools) as it is widely recognized to constitute a significant FCOI. Individuals who serve on speakers' bureaus ...are seen as essential to the marketing of diseases as well as drugs."

There are high threshold limits on money allowed from the industry: $10.000 per year and $50,000 in stock holdings in pharmaceutical companies.

These actions contradict the APA's statement to foster an "unbiased, evidence based DSM free from any conflict of interest."

There are 3 essential goals for the panels of the DSM according to this article:

1. All DSM taskforce members should be free of FCOLs
2. Individuals who have participated in speakers' bureaus should be prohibited from DSM panel participation.
3. Individuals with any association with the industry should not be involved in the decision-making.

10. Criticism of the DSM

Not everybody was happy with the categories in the DSM.

Allen J. Frances, former head of the psychiatry department at Duke University, wrote under "DSM-5 in Distress", posted December 2, 2012: "DSM is a Guide not a Bible - Ignore Its ten worst changes. APA approval of DSM-5 is a sad day for psychiatry."

He claims that the

> "saddest moment" in his 45-year career is the American Psychiatric Association's final approval to a "deeply flawed DSM5(sic) containing many changes that seem clearly unsafe and scientifically unsound."

His best advice to clinicians, the press and the general public:

> "Be skeptical and don't follow DSM 5 blindly down a road likely to lead to massive over-diagnosis and harmful over-medication. Just ignore the ten changes that make no sense."

He states that there were many

> ill-conceived and risky proposals that were opposed by more than fifty mental health professional associations who petitioned for an outside review and independent judgment. Journals, the press, and the public expressed astonishment about some decisions that seemed to lack scientific support and lack of common sense.

He writes that some of the earlier proposals were fortunately dropped, like rape as a mental disorder. He rejects the idea that there are financial ties to pharma, although

> "so many of the DSM changes will enhance pharma profits."

He feels that people working on the DSM-5 did so with "pure hearts". He also points out that 80 % of psychiatric drugs are prescribed in primary care.

In the following, Frances lists what he considers the ten most harmful diagnoses:

1. "DSM will turn temper tantrums into a mental disorder- a puzzling decision based on the work of only one research group...my fear is that it will exacerbate ...the already <u>excessive and inappropriate use of medication in young children. During the past two decades, child psychiatry has already provoked three fads -a tripling of Attention Deficit disorder, a more than 20-times increase in Autistic Disorder and a 40-times increase in childhood Bipolar Disorder.</u>"

He feels that the practitioners and the public should be educated about the "difficulty of accurately diagnosing fad and even more inappropriate medication used in vulnerable children." Frances writes:

2. "Normal grief will become Major Depressive Disorder, thus medicalizing and trivializing our expectable and necessary emotional reactions to the loss of a loved one and substituting pills ...for the deep consolation of family, friends, religion and the resiliency that comes with time and the acceptance of the limitations of life."

3. "The everyday forgetting characteristic of old age will now be misdiagnosed as Minor Neurocognitive Disorder, creating a huge false positive of people who are not at special risk for dementia. Since there is no effective treatment for this condition ... It is a dead loss for many who will be mislabeled."

4. "DSM 5 will likely trigger a fad of Adult Attention Deficit Disorder leading to widespread misuse of stimulant drugs."

5. "Excessive eating 12 times in 3 months is not longer just...gluttony. DSM 5 has ...turned it into a psychiatric illness called Binge Eating Disorder."

6. Changes in DSM 5 of Autism will result in lowered rates – Frances fears a reduction in school services.

7. "First-time substance abusers will lumped in …with hardcore addicts despite their very different treatment needs and the prognosis and the stigma this will cause."

8. "DSM 5 has created a slippery slope by introducing the concept of Behavioral Addictions that eventually can spread <u>to make a mental disorder of everything we like to do a lot.</u> Watch out for careless overdiagnosis of internet and sex addiction and the development of lucrative treatment programs to exploit these new markets."

9. "DSM 5 obscures the already fuzzy boundary between Generalized Anxiety Disorder and the worries of everyday life. Small changes in definition can create millions of anxious new "patients" and expand the already <u>widespread practice of inappropriately prescribing addicting anti-anxiety medications.</u>"

10. "DSM 5 has opened the gate further of the already existing problem of misdiagnosis of PTSD in forensic settings."

Frances continues:

> "Except for autism, all the DSM 5 changes losen diagnosis and threaten to turn our current diagnostic inflation into diagnostic hyperinflation. Painful experience with previous DSMs teaches that <u>anything in the diagnostic system that can be misused and turned into a fad, will be</u>. Many millions of people with normal grief, gluttony, distractibility, worries, reactions to stress, the temper tantrums of childhood, the forgetting of old age and "behavioral addictions" will soon be mislabeled as psychiatrically sick and given inappropriate treatment." He feels that people with real psychiatric problems will be shortchanged.

He closes with:

> <u>"DSM 5 violates the most sacred (and most frequently ignored) tenet in medicine: First Do No Harm! "That's why this is such a sad moment."</u>

Stuart Kirk and Herb Kutchins, professors of social welfare or social work, already criticized the previous edition of DSM-5, namely DSM IV. They state in their book "The selling of DSM " (2008) after confirming that Kraepelin is the basis for the current identification of mental disorders (p.5) that diagnostic reliability is a problem in the previous edition (DSM III).
In their earlier book "Making us crazy" (1997) they wrote:

> "DSM is a claim for professional jurisdiction by the American Psychiatric Association. The broadness of their claim provides justification for the scope of psychiatric expertise and a basis for requests for governmental and private support. But it does more: it proposes how we as a society should think about our trouble." (p.11)

> "The diagnostic manual … is used frequently in the judicial system when questions are raised about a defendant's mental capacity … or cognitive abilities. In legal cases involving guardianship, child custody, criminal liability… testimony about diagnostic categories are frequently invited and the guidelines provided by the DSM are therefore introduced." (p.11)

> "In schools…children who are having problems with their academic work, their peers, their teachers or their families are being labeled by the users of DSM as suffering of disorders…These children may be placed in special classes, dismissed from school or given medication. From prisons to child welfare… agencies, DSM is shaping how we think about problems and determining who gets labeled as having a mental disorder" (p.12)

> "In fact, one of the most powerful effects of DSM is due to its connection to insurance coverage… it is the key to millions of dollars in insurance coverage for psychotherapy, hospitalization and medication." (p12)

Because each mental health professional has to list a psychiatric diagnostic label and code number on their claims for insurance reimbursement not only from private health insurance carriers but also from massive government programs such as Medicaid, Social Security Disability Income, benefits for veterans and Medicare...decisions about which problems get included as mental disorders in DSM and who qualifies for the diagnosable diagnostic label <u>are vulnerable to pressure from advocacy groups , professional associations and corporations."(p.12)</u>

They write:

> "It is well known that drug companies provide substantial funding for the American Psychiatric Association's conventions and major scientific journals. It is less well known that <u>some pharmaceutical companies have contributed directly to the development of the DSM.</u>" (p.13)

The authors describe how a self-checklist (<u>PrimeMD</u>) can help primary care physicians identify anxiety, depression, alcoholism and so on in patients who seek help for the flu etc. <u>Pfizer paid for the development of this list and holds the copy right for it.</u> (p.13) (according to the authors, 6000 doctors use PrimeMD) and explains to doctors how to apply for 3rd party reimbursement. (p. 13,14)

The authors also point out DSM's "enormous impact in the halls of science" (p.14). They claim that

> <u>"any psychiatric researcher who seeks funding from the National Institute of Mental Health (NIMH) must do so by using the DSM categories and definitions.</u>" (p.14).

They claim that the influence on public policy is "more immediate" (p.14):

> "Congress and State legislature use statistics on the number of people in the United States who suffer from mental illness as one basis for allocating public funds to various health programs...To the extent that DSM is flawed, these national counts of the mentally ill are misleading to the public policy makers. The private citizen should also be concerned about the basis for DSM diagnoses...<u>diagnoses</u>

<u>that can be stigmatizing and consequential in ways that are almost impossible for the individual to control" (p.14).</u>

They describe the case of a young lawyer who was involved in an abusive relationship. In order to secure payment from the insurance company, the psychotherapist exaggerated her problem and blamed her for the problem rather than her partner. She was prescribed a psychotropic which she never took:

> "Two years later, she is shocked to learn that she now has a psychiatric history of mental disorder and that her medical records are available to her current (and any future) employer, other insurance companies, the state and just about anyone else who may want to know…This lack of privacy and confidentiality … is a major reason why the public should be concerned about DMS's validity and the accuracy of its use." (p.15).

The authors feel that "DSM oversteps its bounds by defining how we should think about ourselves; how we should respond to stress; how much anxiety or sadness we should feel; and when and how we should sleep, eat and express ourselves sexually." (p.15)
They identify several themes in their book:

1. The "pathologizing" of everyday behavior.
2. The "fragility" of science in the "face of political advocacy"
    They say "We find that political negotiations and advocacy- as well as personal interest – are just as, and often more important in determining whether a mental disorder is created." (p.16)
3. How the DSM can be an "instrument that pathologizes those in our society who are undesirable and powerless." (p.16)

They call mental disorders a "construct", i.e. concepts of something "that is not real in a physical sense, but shared ideas, supported by general agreement." (p.23). They state:

"Be aware that constructs such as <u>Generalized Anxiety Disorder</u> are
held together by agreements and that agreements change over time.
The category itself is an invention, a creation" (p.23) "DSM is a
compendium of constructs." (p.24)

They point out that "the meaning of anxiety-based mental disorder has been
officially changed in DSM three times just since 1979 (p. 24) So, if you were
nervous about speaking in public – there are now 7 categories. They feel that the
constructs keep changing and "multiplying like guppies" (p.25). The authors feel
that there are two problems with the DSM:

1. Diagnosis: Since there are so many labels, it is difficult for experts to
   agree (s. arguments between psychiatrists in the "Tree of Life" (Robert
   Bowers) massacre.)
2. Diagnostic validity: If the threshold is too low, the diagnosis might be
   ridiculed as happened with the inclusion of coffee related disorders.
   (p.27)

The authors also describe how homosexuality was first considered to be a mental
disease but was finally expunged.

At the end of their book they offer several suggestions to remedy the
problems of the DSM:
"DMS should narrow its definitions of mental disorders to those conditions where
there is substantial scientific consensus that there is evidence of an internal
mental dysfunction. We have demonstrated how easily the existing criteria can be
and are misused <u>to label as mentally ill people who are troubled but who
probably have no mental disorder.</u>

1.) DSM and its sponsors should be much more modest in their
    proclamation about the scientific foundations, for the manual DSM's
    definition of mental disorders is <u>flawed</u>, the claims of validity and
    reliability as a manual as a whole are shaky, and the causes of most
    mental disorders are unknown.
2.) Clinicians should use the DSM honestly.

3.) We as society should "develop services to assist troubled children,
adults and families without labelling so many of them as mentally ill. The
public may gain false comfort from a diagnostic psychiatry manual that
encourages belief in the illusion that the harshness, brutality and pain in
their lives and in their communities can be explained by a psychiatric
label and eradicated by a pill. Far too often the psychiatric bible has
been making us crazy- when we are just human." (p. 264, 265.)

Psychologist Gary Greenberg (in his book "The book of Woe" (2013) is also
very critical of the DSM. He states the fact that any psychiatrist will acknowledge
that there are no blood tests or brain scans that prove that there is a mental
disorder. He claims : "Psychiatric diagnosis is fiction, sold to the public as fact"
(p.333) He writes about Allen Frances:

> "He's warned anyone who will listen that the DSM-5 will turn even
> more of our suffering into mental illness and, in turn, into grist for
> the pharmaceutical mill." (p. 22)

He claims that the 150 men and women on the task force to "manufacture fiction
and yet act as if it were fact" (p.25) He also states that there is not one biological
test for a DSM disorder (p. 64) and that the theory of a lack of serotonin has been
"abandoned for lack of evidence"(p. 64). He again cites Allen Frances who even
calls it "diagnostic imperialism" (p. 142) or "psychiatric diagnosis gone wild" (cited
on p.143) or "psychiatrizing normal behavior." (p. 148) He mentions the authors
Wakefield and Horwitz, who state in their book "The Loss of Sadness" (2007) that
psychiatric diagnosis was a potential harm against which we need protection".
(p.162.)

Greenberg cites psychiatrist Ken Kendler who criticizes the fact that the
DSM diagnoses a mental disorder solely by its symptoms:

> "We all know that the DSM is at its best a clumsy and imperfect field
> guide to our foibles and at its worst a compendium of expert
> opinions masquerading as scientific truth... a book whose usefulness
> is primarily commercial "(p.167).

He cites psychologist <u>David Elkins</u>, head of one of the American Psychological Association's divisions who had complained about the DMS' "lowered diagnostic threshold, shay evidence, carelessness with public health." (p.275).

He also mentions psychologist <u>Paula Caplan</u> who had started her own petition, calling for a boycott of the DSM and for congressional hearings into the harmful effects of psychiatric diagnosis."(Greenberg, p.306) Greenberg states: "psychiatric diagnosis is fiction, sold to the public as fact." (p.333). In her book "<u>They say you're crazy</u>" (1995) she had bemoaned the fact that "psychiatrists have nearly unique legal power to prescribe drugs and to order patients committed for treatment against their will." (Caplan, p.29) Like other critics of the DSM she had felt that the psychiatric professionals looked only at the individuals and neglected to consider outside factors like poverty, racism, old age etc. as causes of e.g. depression. She had written:

> "An especially worrisome practice that is on the increase is to assume that a patient who has a physical problem such as stomach pain…must have a mental disorder if physicians have not been able to identify a physiological cause" (Caplan, p.67)

And like her colleagues Kirk and Kutchins, she had stated that "all mental disorders listed in the DSM are constructs."(Caplan, p.193, 194) She had cited these two authors who had claimed

> "No full, comprehensive report with methodological details [of the research of the handbook] was ever made available." (Caplan, p.195)

"In brief, the research shows that DSM's reliability is poor, that two therapists are not impressively likely to assign the same label …to the same person." (p. 203) She again had cited Kirk and Kutchins in "The Selling of DSM":

> "As the evidence makes clear, the DSM players have chosen neither science nor logic – nor very much concern about the harm they do – as grounds for their choices" (Caplan, p.218)

Caplan had claimed that the DSM authors had ignored inquiries, requests for copies, contradicting themselves, lying right out, excluding diagnoses they consider undesirable. She had claimed, that [it] "allows therapists who so wish to sweep far more patients –with their fees into their treatment circle" (p.231) She had cited the psychiatrist <u>Peter Breggin</u> who said:

> "<u>organized psychiatry is big business more than it's a profession. As a big business, managed by APA and NIMH,</u> it develops media relationships, hires PR firms, develops its medical image, holds press conferences to publicise its products, lobbies on behalf of its interests and issues "scientific" reports that protect its members from malpractice suits by lending legitimacy to brain-damaging technologies". (Toxic psychiatry, (1991) p.366-7)

Caplan had stated like many other critics:

> "DSM as a whole discourages practitioners from exploring the social and political environment that causes people pain… I hope that awareness of <u>how the world's most powerful psychiatrists decide who is normal, will sensitize us to the way such judgments are made by and about us in every aspect of our daily lives"</u>. (Caplan, p.274)

She had urged all interested people to "assemble petitions, write letters to experts and the media about what worries you and obtain publicity about the way that judgment about what is normal affects you. Consumers of mental health services now have the legal right in many places to obtain their files, how they have been diagnosed and what their therapists have written about them." (Caplan, p.284.)

Besides Paula Caplan, Greenberg also cites <u>Arnold Relman</u>, MD, former editor of the New England Journal of Medicine, professor emeritus (and husband of Marcia Angell) who said that psychiatric experts lack biological findings that can anchor diagnosis in something beyond symptoms. (p. 334) Greenberg claims that no mental disorder meets scientific demands and he feels that the DSM is "an invented world" and is wrong to characterize psychological suffering as medical illness. (p. 335)

He also cites psychiatrist <u>Thomas Insel,</u> former head of the NIMH, who felt that psychiatrists were "trapped by the DSM. "These [the disorders] are just constructs. There is no reality to schizophrenia or depression." (p.340) Greenberg points out the brain's awe inspiring character, its <u>hundred billions neurons, five hundred trillion synapses, its huge possible</u> <u>connections</u> , is not understood at this point (p.345) He charges that the public is eager to turn over their and their children's troubles to their brain (and to the doctors who claim to understand them) and who are
"quite so willing to gobble down mind- altering medications whose mechanism of action and long-term effects are as unknown as their capacity to blunt feelings is known." (p.345)

He feels that psychiatrists are in the
> "grips of forces bigger than they are ...It's not their fault ...<u>that</u>
> <u>diseases are market opportunities</u>" (p.346).

He writes that the original "healing relationship "must be established in ten-minute medication management visits" (p.347) He also quotes former APA president Paul Fink who answered the question how the diagnosis of bipolar disorder had helped his patient, with: "I got paid." (p. 347). Greenberg cites Kaplan and Sadock, authors of Kaplan and Sadock's "Concise Textbook of Clinical Psychiatry" and he states:
> "they don't mention that there's no reality to those mental disorders
> or warn students of the dangers of reification" (p.347) " even if the
> categories don't exist people can nonetheless be sorted into them."
> (p.348)

He continues citing the authors' text: "Once a diagnosis has been established, a pharmacological treatment strategy can be formulated." (p.348) Greenberg continues: "For bipolar patients the doctor has at her disposal <u>Lithium,</u> anticonvulsants such as <u>Depacote,</u> tranquilizers such as <u>Ativan </u>and antipsychotics such a <u>Haldol</u> and <u>Zyprexa</u>...often it is necessary to try several mood stabilizers before an optimal treatment is found." (p.348)
Greenberg writes:

"more and more people are taking daily doses of drugs whose mechanisms are poorly understood and whose long term consequences are uncertain." (p. 349)

He continues to argue that doctors don't really know if the drug helps you:

"at what cost to the brain, or whether you will be able to stop taking them if you want to nor can they guarantee that you or your child won't become obese or diabetic or die early…"(p.352).

He warns:

"There are undoubtedly patients who would balk. Depressed people might be less willing to surrender their orgasm to Prozac if they don't think they are correcting a biochemical imbalance called Major Depressive Disorder. Psychotic patients might object to a lifetime of taking drugs that blunt their emotions, cloud their cognition, make them gain weight and shorten their life span if they don't think they are being treated for Schizophrenia. Parents might be hesitant to ply their kids with stimulants and antipsychotics if they believe they are merely calming them down rather than treating their ADHD" (p.353).

He states:

"Seventy-two percent of the prescriptions for antidepressants in the United States are written for patients who are not given a psychiatric diagnosis of any kind, who suffer from troubles ranging from tiredness and headaches to "abnormal sensations" and "nonspecific pain". (p. 353)

He wants psychiatrists to admit that they are not sure about the "scientific status" of their diagnostic diagnosis and states:

"The one master to whom we all seem to submit: the market place." (p.355)

He continues:

"We have placed our wellbeing in the not-so-invisible hands of a medical industrial complex whose proprietors have a stake in reducing suffering to biochemistry. It has spawned a psychiatry that can't help giving us more and more diseases."(p.356)

I have already quoted <u>Allan Horwitz,</u> PhD, professor of Sociology at Rutgers University and <u>Jerome Wakefield</u>, PhD, professor of Social Work at New York University. Now I want to quote what they said about the DSM in their book "The Loss of Sadness – how Psychiatry Transformed Normal Sorrow into Depressive Disorder" (2007):

> "One of the most popular theories posits that a chemical imbalance in the brain, specifically deficient amounts of the neurochemical serotonin causes depression. It follows, then, that drug treatments targeting serotonin, the selective serotonin reuptake inhibitors (SSRIs), which presumably correct this chemical imbalance, are the appropriate response to depressive disorders. This theory is relentlessly promoted in many ways: pharmaceutical advertisements emphasize how correctable chemical imbalances cause depressive disorders, public service messages stress that depression stems from flaws in brain chemistry rather than in character, and mental health advocacy groups advance the message that depression is a physical, brain based illness, just like diabetes and asthma. These ubiquitous messages have led to the widespread impression that research has actually shown that chemical deficiencies are the cause of depressive disorders and that drugs work because they correct these impairments in the neurotransmission system. Therefore, it might seem that one way to separate depressive disorders from normal sadness would be to examine levels of serotonin in the brain." (p.168) but "Statements that depression is a "flaw in chemistry" or a "physical disease" are premature; cognitive, psychodynamic, social or other factors...may well cause at least some depressive disorders." (p. 170)

The authors conclude that brain researchers "fail to consider the context in which sadness develops, they are in danger of misdiagnosing the normally sad as having depressive disorders" (p. 177). They continue (in regard to the DSM-III):

> "Pharmaceutical companies were best able to capitalize on the DSM's focus on symptoms, which allowed them to broadly construe states of intense sadness as depressive disorder and thus to <u>vastly increase the potential market for antidepressant medication.</u>"(p. 179).
> "The diagnosis of Major Depression which used common symptoms such as sadness, lack of energy, or sleeplessness as indicators was particularly well suited for expanding the market for psychotropic drugs because it inevitably encompassed many patients who formerly might have been thought to be suffering from problems of living." (p.182)

The authors state:

> "The influence of the pharmaceutical industry is considerable and now extends well beyond the specific promotion of drugs. It donates substantial amounts of money to patient and family advocacy groups that promote the view that depression is a chemical deficiency to be remedied through the use of drugs. These companies also sponsor widespread educational campaigns, such as <u>National Depression Awareness Day</u>, which offer free screening for depression in universities and hospitals. In addition, they provide 800 numbers and Internet screening sites that allow responders to make self-diagnoses of depression and that urge them to consult their physicians to obtain prescriptions for the companies' products. Drug companies also fund the screening efforts in primary medical care and schools...Moreover, the pharmaceutical industry sponsors a considerable proportion of clinical research on depression; <u>the discipline of psychiatry itself is now thoroughly enmeshed with the corporate culture of this industry.</u> Industry-academics collaborations are becoming increasing sources of funding for universities, academic medical centers and hospitals." (p. 187)

> "Now… the legitimacy that the DSM concept of depression accords to
> the widespread treatment of common symptoms of normal malaise
> has become so entrenched that these groups have come to accept a
> definition of depressive disorder that encompasses much normal
> sadness and to endorse the use of antidepressant medications to
> deal with such conditions. (p.188)

The authors list arguments against using anti-depressants. One argument is, that they

> treat as pathological what is "actually an inherent and valuable part
> of the human condition…Using pills represents an escape from truly
> confronting life's problems." (p.190).

Another argument is that it "leads people to accept, rather than resist, oppressive situations…[and] misconstrues social problems as personal problems." (p.190) and they cite a former General Surgeon General, L.E. Burney who had warned in 1985 "that problems of daily living "cannot be "solved with a pill". (cited on p. 190)

Another concern that was raised was

> "whether normal emotions of sadness are a legitimate subject for
> public concern or, instead, a personal matter…<u>Private selves become
> increasingly available for public scrutiny and regulation through
> screening and subsequent medication. The detection of emotions
> and feelings is inevitably far more intrusive and coercive than is the
> detection of physical diseases that usually do require
> help.</u>"(p.190/191).

The authors continue with the next argument which questions the drugs' effectiveness and safety. They claim that their side effects like loss of sexual desire, nausea, diarrhea and headaches are more common and malignant than their advocates claim. (p.191). They also cite the danger of heightened occurrence of suicide, although, they say, that this claim is not "well established", and they point out the uncertainty of long-term use.

They also emphasize that there is no evidence that these medications are more effective than placebos. They cite (p. 191) the Medical Research Council trial and the early National Institute for Health trial. They also quote a comprehensive review by the National Institute for Health and Clinical Excellence (NICE) in England "that suggests that

> SSRIs do not have clinically meaningful advantages over placebos across the entire range of severity of conditions."

A report on this study concluded: "Given doubts about their benefits and concerns about their risks current recommendations for prescribing antidepressants should be reconsidered."(p.191)

The authors do not condemn generally the use of antidepressants and feel that they might be helpful in the hands of a capable physician for patients who are "truly depressed."(p.192)

Another critic, Peter Conrad, professor of Social Sciences at Brandeis University, writes in his book "The Medicalization of Society" (2007) that the number of life problems that are defined as medical, have grown immensely. He feels that

> "life's problems have now received medical diagnoses and are subject to medical treatment despite dubious evidence of their medical nature." (p.3)

and that

> "the long-influential pharmaceutical companies comprise America's most profitable industry." (p.15)

He continues: "In psychiatry… the focus [shifted]… from psychotherapy and family interaction to psychopharmacology, neuroscience and genomics. This shift will be enforced when third –party payers will pay for drug treatments but severely limit individual and group therapies. The choice available to many doctors and patient-consumers is not whether to have talking or pharmaceutical therapies, but rather which brand of drugs should be prescribed" (p.15) He points out that there is a widespread corporatization of healthcare and also, that the Food and Drug Administration Modernization Act (FDAMA) made several changes that have facilitated medicalization. "[It] loosened the restrictions placed on the kind of information that pharmaceutical companies could share with physicians regarding "off-label uses of their drugs" (p.16) As a consequence the

> "amount of information that must be included in the DTC (direct-to-consumer advertising) has decreased."(p.19)

When the FDA approves a drug it can only be advertised for a specific disease and age group for which it was tested, but doctors can use it for any disease. ("off – label"). "Pharmaceutical companies can give doctors information about off-label use as long as they can provide doctors with adequate scientific information or were engaged in clinical trials for the new use." (p.16,17) Risks were not mentioned, but websites could be accessed. He cites Paxil's program director, Barry Brand:

> "Every marketer's dream is to find an unidentified or unknown market and develop it. That's what we were able to do with social anxiety disorder."(SAD) (p.18).

 Conrad states that the sale of Paxil (also for generalized anxiety disorder) (GAD) has been "extremely successful." (p.19) However, in 2002, a federal judge ordered a temporary halt to Paxil ads because it was found that it is habit-forming contrary to the claims of the company and that it may increase the risk of suicide in adolescents. (it has been banned for children and adolescents in the UK along with other SSRIs). In Conrad's words "Companies are now marketing diseases, not just drugs." (p.19) He mentions as an example the medicalization of alcoholism that now includes adult children of alcoholics, enablers and codependents, (p.119), obesity and aging. There is an

> "increasing medical jurisdiction over the whole process of aging – from minor memory deficits to mobility limits to the process of dying." (p.120).

Conrad also examines ADHD. He notes the increase in diagnoses. In 1994-1996 there were 2.6 million children diagnosed, from 2000 -2002 that number rose to 5 million. That goes along with an estimated 700 percent increase in prescriptions of stimulant medications in the 1990s. (p.127). Conrad writes:

"While stimulants like <u>Ritalin</u> and newer drugs like <u>Concerta</u> and <u>Adderall</u> had been approved for the use with children, <u>few of the widely used antidepressants, especially the Selective Serotonin Reuptake Inhibitors (SSRIs) had FDA approval for the use with children under the age of 18.</u>

But physicians can approve such drugs, approved for adults, for children on an off-label basis. He notes that

> "one fifth of individuals who... received a prescription for psychotropics had no mental health diagnosis."

He also notes that 10 % of adolescents who visit a doctor's office receive a psychotropic medication (in the year 2000 to 2001). He further points out that there has been concern about the overuse of psychotropics among children and adolescents, resulting in suicide and excess deaths (p.129) which prompted the British medical authorities to ban SSRIs for children and the FDA to add a black box warning to the medication. He feels that there is an

> "increased medicalization of the social and emotional difficulties in adolescents. Problems that a decade ago would not have been appropriate for medication are now managed with psychotropics, even apparently sometimes without any mental health diagnosis" (p.129)

The author mentions reports of studies suggesting that half of all Americans will become mentally ill. He names in particular the 2001-3 National Comorbidity Survey (NCSR) (p.130). It is based on a survey of 9000 respondents aged 18 -54 with the "stunning" findings that nearly half the population will, according to the DSM-IV, have a diagnosable mental disorder in their lifetime. Conrad states that there are several ways to interpret these findings, among others, sadness. Therefor they include all symptoms of sadness under depression and therefore overestimate the prevalence of mental disorders.

This encourages the medicalization of everyday troubles and suggests that a hugely wide range of behaviors have to be included to cover such a large population and that the gap between a mild disorder and normal life difficulties is very narrow. He claims: "While there are undoubtedly people with serious disorders who are untreated, just as likely there are people with mild problems who are diagnosed, most likely with psychotropic medications." (p.130) He continues

> "Without being too cynical, one could say this study is a <u>boon for the drug companies;</u> consider the yet untapped market for their products." (p.130)

Conrad criticizes that in surveys the research interviewer completely ignored context or history of the individual. (p.131) They make, e.g. no difference between a person being sad about the death of a loved one or being generally depressed and they suggest psychiatric treatment as their solution. This approach aligns or perhaps encourages the enormous rise over the past decade in "the use of psychotropic medications for an increasing range of problems."

> "It will be interesting to see if the current concern with suicide risks among adolescents taking SSRIs or that the recent reports of increased cardiac risks from stimulants will have an impact on the number of individuals who receive treatments with these drugs"(p.132)

Conrad is taking a closer look at the drug <u>Paxil</u> and states: "It is clear that GlaxoSmithKline's campaign for Paxil increased the medicalization of anxiety, implying that shyness and worrying may be a medical problem with Paxil as the proper treatment." (p. 135)

Other medications Conrad examines more closely are psychotropic drugs for children. To cite him:

> "<u>Children's problems constitute a growing market for psychotropic drugs</u>"(p.135)

"Marketing diseases and then promoting drugs to treat those diseases is now common practice in the pharmaceutical world made all the more lucrative with DTC. (Direct to Consumer Advertising) "(p.135)

Conrad warns of non-profit consumer groups like CHADD or the National Alliance for the Mentally Ill (NAMI) who "have become strong supporters for medical treatment for the human problems for which they advocate". (p.139) Both receive financial support, in NAMI's case $12 million from pharmaceutical companies (source cited on p.140) ...raising the question of where consumer advocacy begins and pharmaceutical promotion ends." (p.140) (There are Internet sites that warn of the danger of psychotropics like the "Alliance for Human Research Protection" (www. ahrp.org.)) (The aim of this group is ethical medical research to protect human rights, welfare and dignity. The group's founder, Vera Sharav, became active after her son, who had been diagnosed with schizo-affective disorder and prescribed Clozapine, died after taking this medication. (Wikipedia, Nov. 28, 2023)]

Conrad continues:

> "Drug companies are having an increasing impact on the boundaries of the normal and the pathological, becoming active agents of social control" (p.143) and may feel more responsible to shareholders than patients.

He also feels that by treating e.g. a child simply by his or her symptoms instead of examining the social context and dealing with problems in society, those problems are ignored or pushed aside.

He claims:" Medicalization is prevalent in the United States but is increasingly an international phenomenon" (p.144) facilitated by multinational drug companies.

Prior to the publication, critics of the DSM-5 developed and circulated a petition that was sponsored and signed by many mental health organizations that called for an outside review of the document.("Mental Health", Nov. 15, 2013)

I want to name a few more critical voices:

The Lancet, the highly regarded English medical journal, wrote in an editorial in May 11, 2013 under the title "Bipolar disorder at the extreme :"

> "to critics, the growth of the diagnostic manual- still based on subjective observation-represents an illusion of precision and, at worst, pathologizes normal human experiences."

<u>Awais Aflab</u>, MD, writes under the title "Conceptualization of Mental Illness and Historical Evolution of Pychiatric Classification (RC Psych Webinar, August 26,2021):

> "In mental health, we are stymied by our language. The most obvious linguistic problem can be found in our current diagnostic terms what my predecessor Steve Hyman has called "fictive" categories. Terms outstrips their scientific value. Each refers to a cluster of symptoms...there should be no presumption that these are singular disorders, each with a single cause and a common treatment."

<u>Thomas Insel</u>, former director of the NIMH, writes:

> "Classification based on the Kraepelinian system have continued to be used in some form or other all over the world. Many psychiatrists have done so under protest and expressed their disbelief in the working hypothesis underlying that system." (in : Erwin Stengel, 1958, "DSM III [is] deeply imbedded in implicit neo-Krapelian assumption.")

<u>Kupfer, First and Regier</u> state in „Research Agenda for DSM IV 2002":"Any of the DSM-defined symptoms'...lack of treatment specific is the rule rather than the exception"

The psychiatrist Dr. Paniagua warns us not to identify cultural issues with mental illness. As an example, cultures are listed that reward interdependence amid family members. This should not be confused with separation anxiety or the refusal to speak a new language as selective mutism.

Lindsey Hoeschen writes in "Neo-Kraepellian Divergence, from Kraepelin , what are they and why do they matter." (Undergraduate Honors Thesis, Portland State University). She writes about ADHD:

> "3 %of adults met the criteria for the condition, 84.1 % of this population were also diagnosed with mood disorders...There was a significant increase in the diagnosis of adult ADHD in 2002 after a new drug had been marketed in the US to treat the symptoms. If a specific drug worked for a certain condition, it would prove some justification for the diagnosis. This is not the case. The treatment only

eliminates symptoms. There are no objective tests. Modern diagnosis practices based on the DSM not only bypass the individual and environmental and makes definite diagnoses on the symptoms alone. [They] are often followed by unjustified prescription of medication. They are unjustified, because their employment alone presumes a biological cause correctable with a specific kind of medication without these being a known biological cause."

So only the symptoms are treated masking and allowing any underlying mechanisms to continue. The idea of any other medical discipline practicing this way is almost unimaginable. In the absence of objective tests which validate suspected diagnoses by detecting underlying biological causes, psychiatric diagnoses are subjectively made on the basis of interpreted signs and symptoms alone. As of today, only 3 % of psychiatric conditions have been causally established (Stevenson)... ground psychiatry on valid and reliable bases comparable to other medical disciplines ...the diagnosis must be validated by objective tests." Most diagnosed mental health conditions are treated based on consensus guidelines and FDA –approved medication therapy. It is important to note that none of the disorders can be shown to have a physical cause – they cannot be shown to show a chemical "imbalance", which is a basic requirement for any scientific work as the scientist Candace Pert pointed out. Pert felt that

> If you can't measure something, you cannot base scientific findings on it.

The treatment does not cure the cause (since there is no proof of the cause), only assumptions, like it is assumed that there is a chemical imbalance. So only the symptoms are being treated and they are treated with very potent medication that involve a lot of problems as we will see later.

Hannah Decker points out in her article "Emil Kraepelin-How Kraepelinian was Kraepelin?" (s. a.)that Kraepelin felt himself that nothing holy was in his nosology (classification) He even doubted the division between manic depressive illness and schizophrenia. He also thought that there were "no fixed, but only blurred borders between mental health and mental illness." (s. a.) She writes "His legacy is balanced on shaky empirical foundation."

Following these points, I want to take a closer look at one of the disorders, ADHD, because I have a great concern for the children and adolescents in the U.S. who take drugs for this disorder.

11. ADHD according to the DSM

(listed under Neurodevelopment Disorders in the DSM-5)(Is it really a faulty development of nerves as they claim? (s. the following FDA statement.)

The FDA states:

"Specific etiology of this symptom is unknown and there is no single diagnostic test" (https://www.accessdata.fda.gov.>drugsatfda_docs.)

The DSM defines the disorder in the following way:

A. "Persistent pattern of inattention and/or hyperactivity – impulsivity that interferes with functioning or development as characterized by 1) inattention and/or 2) hyperactivity and impulsivity.
Note: The symptoms are not solely a manifestation of oppositional behavior.
(My comment: To examine the statement above logically, it says: "Inattention and hyperactivity/impulsivity… [is] characterized by inattention and hyperactivity!" Circular reasoning!
In regard to note: "not solely "does not make any sense –it means it is partly a manifestation of oppositional behavior – what they mean is that it is not! The wordsmiths have to work a little harder!)

There are 6 symptoms listed: (I abbreviated these)

a. Often failure of close attention, careless mistakes
b. Often difficulties to sustain attention (e.g. during lengthy reading)
c. Often does not seem to listen when spoken to even in the absence of any obvious distraction.
d. Often fails to finish schoolwork etc.
e. Often has difficulty organizing tasks
f. Often avoids, dislikes or is reluctant to engage in tasks that require sustained mental effort
g. Often loses things

h. Often easily distracted by external stimuli (for older adolescents and adults may include unrelated thoughts) Often forgetful in daily activities (e.g. doing chores)

There are several unscientific expressions here:
    1.) What does "often" mean?
    2.) What does "seem" (c) mean?

To summarize: The disorders mentioned here, are:

No close attention
No sustained attention
No listening
No finishing of work
Not good at organizing work
Reluctance to engage in tasks
Losing things
Forgetfulness

Organizing these "disorders", we basically have 3:

Distractibility
Poor organization skills
Reluctance to work

The classifications for hyperactivity and impulsivity:
Fidgets
Leaves seat
Runs about
Unable to play
Often "on the go"
Talks excessively
Blurts out answers
Often has troubles waiting his turn
Interrupts

There are different combinations of both groups of symptoms. There is a caveat: these symptoms characterize ADHD, unless "Symptoms are not better explained by another mental disorder" which demonstrates how shaky and unscientific the identification of symptoms is. There are 3 forms:

Mild: "Few, if any symptoms in excess of those required to make the diagnosis…"
Moderate: "Between minor and severe…"
Severe: "Many symptoms in excess of those required to make the diagnosis…"
(By the way, I am sure that there are disorders where the child runs around and can't be stopped – I witnessed a child like that in a train in Europe, but I believe that the child had a neurological disorder that could be proven. As one scientist stated (s. a.) "You can only prove something if you can count it.")

What is ignored in these classifications are the problems of poor parenting (e.g. not sending kids to bed on time), poverty, poor nutrition, poor teaching techniques (like block classes, no change in presentation) etc.
Many people are "guilty" of the listed "disorders. The many self-help-books attest to that. (Who has not "listened" to a sermon and thought about a dress or hat that one of the parishioners wore!)

I looked at the guidance concerning ADHD that is given to school counselors: "hyperactivity, distractibility, or impulsivity are present in all children to some degree. When children demonstrate these behaviors more than do their peers, however, the problem could be ADHD." (Resources for working with children with attention –deficit/hyperactivity disorder(ADHD) JR Lucker, AT Molloy. Elementary School Guidance and counseling, 1995. JSTOR. (stands for Journal storage, "provided full-text searches of almost 2,000 journals." (Wikipedia, June 15, 24)

Since there is no chemical proof of this disorder the term "more than do their peers" is highly unscientific. It ignores many factors like average class behavior, teacher style (I have seen teachers who accept very undisciplined behavior like walking around, interrupting etc. If students see this in their peers they pick up these behaviors.)

12. Description of ADHD and side effects of Ritalin on the PPI

 With a diagnosis of ADHD, the drug most often prescribed, is, as I have stated, Ritalin. (Methylphenidate Hydrochloride). I decided to take a look at the patient packet insert (PPI), the paper that is given to you when you pick up your medication. I was interested to find out who wrote these pamphlets and I found out that they are submitted to the FDA voluntarily by the manufacturers and then approved by the FDA. I examined a pamphlet that had the code Code-1-020, Rev 5/91. As you might expect, the print is in small letters, the language used is vague and deceiving and sounds positive and for many terrible side effects medical terms are used that, I am sure, the layman doesn't know and does not look up. The description starts with:

> "(Methylphenidate Hydrochloride) is a mild central nervous system stimulant. The mode of action in man is not completely understood…There is neither specific evidence which clearly establishes the mechanism whereby methylphenidate produces its mental and behavioral effects in children nor conclusive evidence regarding how these effects relate to the condition of the central nervous system… Specific etiology of this syndrome (ADHD) is unknown and there is no single diagnostic test…Sufficient data on safety and efficacy of long-term use …are not yet available. Although a causal relationship has not been established, suppression of growth has been reported with long-term use of stimulants in children. "

In plain language:

- The medication is "mild" although when you read the list of adverse reactions following, you can hardly call it that.
- The manufacturers don't know how it works.
- There is no evidence that it works.
- It is not known what ADHD is and there are no tests for it.
- It is not known if the medication is safe or effective.
- Sufficient data …of long-term use are not yet available.

(The wordsmiths did a wonderful job with the PPI!)

Listed adverse reactions in the PPI:

Nervousness and insomnia are the most common reactions, then there are

- Hypersensitivity (skin rash, urticarial = skin condition that causes itchy welts)
- Fever
- Arthralgia (joint pain)
- Exfoliative dermatitis
- Erythema multiforme with histopathological findings of necrotizing vasculitis (this is an infection, leads to inflammation of blood vessels that can cause tissues to die, can lead to death in a matter of hours. (according to Johns Hopkins: medicine)
- Thrombocytopenic purpura (blood disorder that can be characterized by a decrease in the number of platelets in the blood)
- Anorexia
- Nausea
- Dizziness
- Palpitations
- Headache
- Dyskinesia (involuntary, erratic body movements)
- Drowsiness
- Blood pressure and pulse changes
- Tachycardia (heartbeat of over a hundred beats a minute)
- Leukopenia (low white blood cell count)
- Angina
- Cardiac arrhythmia
- Tourette syndrome
- <u>Toxic psychosis</u>

Overdoses can lead to convulsions ("Maybe followed by coma.")

According to <u>"Statista"</u> (April 24, 2024) the CDC (Center for Disease Control and Prevention), a government entity, data from 2016-2019 show the following numbers for children and adolescents who have been diagnosed with ADHD:

3-5 years old	2%
6-11 years old	10 %
12-17 years old	13 %

It is difficult for me to see how a dangerous medication like Ritalin can be legally prescribed in our country just to possibly have a lively, curious child "pay attention". And to diagnose and prescribe medication for this to children 3-5 years old!

 In the following, I list other psychotropic drugs that are also often used for children and adolescents and I quote what the FDA says about them.

13. Psychotropic medications approved for ADHD and other mental health disorders for children by FDA and warnings by the FDA, DEA and NIMH

(http://reference.medscape.com/drugs/psychiatric)

<u>Psychotropic drugs</u>

I list them in the same order they appear in the FDA list and I will add the same warning that the FDA gives:

($<$ means younger than, $>$ older than)

ANTIDEPRESSANTS:

         for

- Prozac — MDD, OCD
- Luvox — OCD $<$ 8 years: "Safety and efficacy not established"
- Zoloft — OCD $<$ 6 years: "Safety and efficacy not established"
- Lexapro — MDD
- Elavil — Depression
- Anafranil — OCD $<$ 10 years : "Safety and efficacy not established"
- Norpramine — OCD $<$ 12 years: "Safety and efficacy not established"
- Vivactil — Depression $<$ 12 years: "Safety and efficacy not established"
- Surmontil — Depression $<$ 12 years: "Safety and efficicacy not established"

ANTIPSYCHOTIC AGENTS:

- Abilify — Schizophrenia, Bipolar Mania.
  Tourette Disorder$<$ 6 years: "Safety and efficacy not established"
- Haldol — Schizophrenia, Psychosis/Sedation" $<$3 years: "Safety and efficacy not established"
  Tourette disorder: $<$3 years: "Safety and efficacy not established"

Behavioral Disorders: < 3 years :"Safety and efficacy not established"

Acute Agitation<12 years: "Safety and efficacy not established"

- Navane
- Orap   Tourette Disorder < 2 years: "Safety and efficacy not established"

- Trilafon   Schizophrenia
- Stelacine   Schizophrenia/Psychosis <6 years: "Safety and efficacy not established"

- Saphris   Bipolar Disorder <10 years :"Safety and efficacy not established"

- Invega   Schizophrenia <12 years old:"Safety and efficacy not established"

- Zyprexa   Bipolar I Disorder /Schizophrenia < 13 years "Safety
  and   efficacy not established"
- Seroquel   Schizophrenia <12 years:"Safety and efficacy not established"

  Bipolar I disorder/Mania <10 years "Safety and efficacy not established"

- Risperdal   Schizophrenia < 13 years: "Safety and efficacy not established"

  Bipolar Mania < 10 years "Safety and efficacy not established"

  Autism: Irritability with autistic disorder in children 5-16 years: < 5 years: "Safety and efficacy not established"

- Thorazine   " Behavioal Disorders, Hyperactivity"< 6 months: "Safety and efficacy not established"

  (Can be given to children after 6 moth of age!!!!)

- Compazine   Psychotic Disorder
- Mellaril   Schizophrenia: <2 years: "Safety and efficacy not established"

(Can be given to children after 2 years of age!)

ADHD AGENTS, like STIMULANTS (AMPHETAMINES)

- Adderall   for ADHD, < 3, not recommended. (Can be started at age 3 (!!!)
- Adzenys XR   ADHD: <3 years "Safety and efficacy not established" (Can be given to children after 3 years of age!)
- Ritalin   ADHD : < 3 years:"Safety and efficacy not established"
- Strattera
- Catapres   < 6 years :"not established"
- Dexetrine   <3 years"Safety and efficacy not established" (Can be given to children after 3 years of age!)
- Focalin   < 6 years "Safety and efficiency not established"
- Intuniv   "Safety and efficiency not established"
- Vivanse
- Effexor

ANTIANXIETY AGENTS

- Librium   Anxiety, <6 years "Safety and efficacy not established"
- Valium   "potentially toxic dose in patients > 6 years"
- Metrobamate   <6 years: "Not recommended"
- Serax   <6 years: "Not recommended"
- Cymbalta   < 7 years"Safety and efficiency not established"
- Narcan

SEDATIVES/HYPNOTICS

- Amytal

STIMULANTS

- Desoxyn   <6 years"Safety and efficacy not established"

- Dietylpropio   <16 years: "Safety and efficiency not established"
- Provigil   <16 years: "Not recommended"
- Cafcit   <12 years: "Not recommended"

ADHD garners by far most medications. Each medication lists a name, but there are many other varieties of this medication.

The Food and Drug Administration published the following <u>warnings</u> in the following article:

<u>Suicidality in children and Adolescents Being treated with **Antidepressant Medication**</u>

On February 5, the <u>FDA</u> directed all manufacturers of all antidepressants to revise their labelling by adding a boxed warning and extended warning statements to alert health care providers to an <u>increased risk of suicidal</u> <u>thinking and behavior in children and adolescents who are treated with these antidepressants</u> and to include information about pediatric studies. The FDA has informed the manufacturers that it decided that a Med Guide (Patient Medication Guide) will be given to each patient who takes these drugs to advise them of risks and precautions they may want to take. These labelling changes were made after recommendations by the <u>Psychopharmacologic Drugs Advisory Committee and the Pediatric Drugs Advisory Committee on September 13-14, 2004.</u>
The risks of suicidality were identified in placebo-controlled trials that lasted 4 months. Nine drugs were examined, including the SSRIs which were prescribed for children and adolescents with psychiatric disorders. There were 24 trials involving 4400 patients. The risk for suicidality for patients on these drugs was 4%, vs. placebo risk of 2% (No suicides occurred during the testing.) The FDA decided to include the following points in the boxed warnings:

- Risk of suicidality
- For clinical use this risk must be balanced with the clinical need.

- Patients on these medications should be observed for this risk, for <u>clinical worsening or unusual changes in behavior.</u>
- Families and caregivers should closely observe the patient and communicate with the prescriber.
- A statement as to whether a drug is approved for any pediatric use and if so, which one.

Pediatric patients should be closely observed for <u>clinical worsening, agitation, irritability, suicidality and unusual changes in behavior or at times of dose changes.</u>

The FDA has included the following drugs that should include these warnings:

Anafranil	Paxil
Aventyl	Pexeva
Celexa	Prozac
Cymbalta	Remeron
Desyrel	Sarafem
Effexor	Serzone
Elavyl	Sinequan
Lexapro	Surmontil
Limbitrol	Symbiax
Ludiomil	Tofranil
Luvox	Tofranil PM
Marplan	Triavil
Nardil	Norpramin
Vivactil	Wellbutrin
Pamelo	Zoloft
Parnate	Zyban

On its website the **FDA** warns of side effects of **stimulants** (website, see above): This government entity suggests that

patients being considered for treatment should have a thorough examination for <u>heart related diseases</u> in themselves or their family...Patients who develop symptoms ...of cardiac disease during stimulant treatment should undergo a prompt cardiac evaluation."

<u>Psychiatric Adverse Events:</u> The FDA warns that "stimulants may exacerbate symptoms in "patients with preexisting psychotic disorders..." but also warns of new psychotic or manic symptoms:

<u>Emergence of New Psychotic or Manic Symptoms:</u>

"...psychotic or manic symptoms, e.g. hallucinations, delusional thinking or mania in children or adolescents <u>without prior history of psychotic illness...can be caused by stimulants at usual doses</u>. IF SUCH SYMPTOMS OCCUR, CONSIDERATION SHOULD BE GIVEN TO A POSSIBLE CAUSAL ROLE IN THE STIMULANT, and discontinuation of treatment may be appropriate."

The following are more detailed **warnings by the FDA:**

<u>Aggression:</u> "Aggressive behavior or hostility is often observed in children and adolescents with ADHD and has been reported in clinical trials and the post marketing experience of some medications indicated for the treatment of ADHD...patients beginning treatment for ADHD should be monitored for the <u>appearance of or worsening of aggressive behavior or hostility.</u>"

<u>Long-Term Suppression of Growth:</u> There is a suggestion "that consistently medicated children have a temporary slowing in growth rate <u>without evidence of rebound during this period of development</u>... therefore <u>patients who are not growing or gaining weight as expected may need to have their treatment interrupted.</u>"

<u>Seizures:</u>   "There is some clinical evidence that <u>stimulants may lower the convulsive threshold</u>...very rarely, in patients without a history of

seizures…In the presence of seizures the drug should be
discontinued.

<u>Peripheral Vasculopathy, Including Raynaud's Phenomenon</u>: "Stimulants,
including Adderall, used to treat ADHD are associated with [these
diseases]…very rare sequelae included digital ulceration and/or soft
tissue breakdown…Careful observation for digital changes is
necessary. Effects [of the above diseases] were observed …at
therapeutic doses in all age groups…Careful observation for digital
changes is necessary…Further clinical observation (e.g.,
rheumatology referral) may be appropriate for certain patients."

<u>Serotonin Syndrome</u> basically happens when there is too much serotonin in the
body (this can happen because the reuptake that occurs naturally, is
inhibited by medication, the SSRIs, see a later chapter), because of a
combination with other SSRIs. The FDA : [This is]<u>"a potentially life-
threatening reaction</u> … In these situations, consider an alternative
non-serotonergic drug."
"Serotonin syndrome symptoms <u>may include mental status changes</u>
instability (e.g. tachycardia, labile blood pressure, dizziness,
diaphoresis, flushing, hyperthermia), neuromuscular symptoms
(e.g. agitation, hallucinations, delirium and coma, autonomic
tremor, rigidity, myoclonus, hyperreflexia, incoordination), seizures,
and/or gastrointestinal symptoms (e.g., nausea, vomiting, diarrhea)"

<u>Visual Disturbances</u>: "Difficulties with accommodation and blurring of vision have
been reported with stimulant treatment"

<u>Tics:</u>   "Amphetamines have been reported to <u>exacerbate motor and phonic
tics and Tourette's syndrome</u>… clinical evaluation [for these] should
precede use of stimulant medication."

The FDA adds the following:
          <u>Information for patients:</u>

"Prescribers or other health professionals should inform patients, their families and their caregivers about the benefits and risks associated with treatment with amphetamine or dextroamphetamines and should counsel them in its appropriate use. A patient Medication Guide is available for Adderall."
The FDA urges health professionals to instruct patients, their families and caregivers to discuss the contents of this guide and to obtain answers.

And what does the **DEA** (Department of Justice/United States Drug Enforcement Administration), a government entity, say about **amphetamines (stimulants)**? (under drug fact sheet):

"What is their effect on the body? Similar to cocaine, but slower onset and longer duration, increased body temperature, blood pressure and pulse, insomnia, loss of appetite, physical exhaustion. Chronic abuse produces a psychosis that resembles schizophrenia: paranoia, hallucinations, violent and erratic behavior.

What does the **NIH**, a U.S. Government entity, say about the effects of **sedatives?**

Short term symptoms of use:
Drowsiness
Sedation
slurred speech
Poor concentration
Confusion
Dizziness
Clammy skin
Impaired judgment, coordination and memory
Reduced anxiety (?)
Lowered blood pressure
Slowed breathing

Long-term consequences are: increased risk of respiratory distress

They name, among others: Nembutal, Luminal, Xanax, Limbitrol, Valium, Ativan, Halicon, Lunesta, Sonata, Ambien.

The **DEA** (United States Drug Enforcement Administration) lists 5 groups of substances (schedules) that are essential for law enforcement. Let's look at Schedule II.

Schedule II: Drugs with a high potential for abuse [and] ... and psychological and physical dependence. <u>These drugs are also considered dangerous.</u> (e.g. Methamphetamine, Methadone, Demerol, <u>Dexedrine, Adderall, Ritalin.</u>

Let's take a look at the warning the **FDA** issues for some well known psychotropic medications (<u>https://www.accessdata.fda.gov.>drugsatfda docs</u>.) As of March 2012) Most of them are stimulants (amphetamines) The FDA approves some of them starting at the age 3-6 years, most at the age of 6 years, but also includes the following <u>warnings:</u>

<u>Celexa</u> (Citalopram)	Is an SSRI, <u>can be fatal</u>, should be avoided. "In 3 additional placebo controlled in depressed patients...<u>the difference between patients receiving Celexa and patients receiving a placebo was not statistically different.</u>"
<u>Effexor</u>	<u>Can cause mania, suicidal thinking</u>. <u>Side effects</u>: Anxiety, agitation, panic attacks..., irritability, <u>hostility, aggressiveness</u>, psychomotor restlessness
<u>Luvox</u>:	Can cause, among others, anxiety, agitation, panic attacks, <u>hostility, aggression, increase in suicidal thinking</u>
<u>Prozac</u>	SSRI

Side effects: Mania, seizures, anxiety, potential for cognitive and motor impairment, suicidal thoughts and behavior. Can cause serotonin syndrome when used with other serotonergic agents (other antidepressants or herbs.)

Ritalin   SSRI

Suitable for pediatric patients 6 years and older

Side effects: Serious cardiovascular events, may cause psychotic or manic symptoms in patients with no prior history of symptoms like hallucinations and delusional thinking, painful prolonged penile erection, long-term suppression of growth, anxiety, insomnia, abdominal pain

Seroquel   for bipolar disorder, efficacy was established in 2 twelve week monotherapy trials

Side effects: Suicidal thoughts or behavior, tardive dyskinesia, potential for cognitive and motor impairment, abnormal thinking (p.27).

Xanax   Antianxiety

Side effects: Seizures after withdrawal, mania, suicide

Zoloft   SSRI, for, among others, PTSD

Side effects: Suicidal thoughts and behavior, difficulty concentrating, confusion, unsteadiness

Let's pause for a moment: Children, sometimes as young as three, are prescribed medication for inattention and forgetfulness with drugs that can cause severe physical impairments, addiction and mental ailments like hallucinations, delusional thinking or mania (according to warnings from the FDA.) and they can get entrapped into a treatment cycle where they end up getting treated for symptoms that are caused by the drugs they take. (That explains why some children and adolescents are treated with several, sometimes up to fourteen different psychotropic drugs.)

It is ironic that a nurse who recently forged a signature on a prescription for morphine cream (0.1% morphine cream) was charged with a felony count of prohibited acts etc. as reported in the Tribune Review on Jan. 29, 2024. The author of the article writes:

> "The cream is a schedule II controlled substance…According to the DEA, schedule II substances are drugs with a high potential for abuse with use potentially leading to severe psychological or physical dependence. They include [among others] Adderall and Ritalin."

It is sad that we allow our children to be treated with these dangerous medications that may send a grown-up to prison for using them, just to increase their attention span in class!

Because Ritalin is such a popular drug to treat ADHD I want to take a closer look at this psychotropic medication.

14. Ritalin

Ritalin, an SSRI, was created in Switzerland. It is primarily used for ADHD, but also for depression and other mental disorders. It affects the brain function and is a stimulant. The Drug Enforcement Administration (DEA) classified it as a Schedule 2 narcotic (s. a.), the same classification given to cocaine, morphine and amphetamines. At this time there are about 10 % of children, mostly boys, on this medication. (s. chapter 12) The DSM IV stated concerning Ritalin: "There are no laboratory tests that have been established as diagnostic in the clinical assessment of [ADHD]. "(The New American/ June 10, 1996.)

Psychologist John Rosemond states in regard to Ritalin:

> "(a) no biological anomaly has been found to be reliably associated with any psychiatric diagnosis

> (b) no one has ever quantified the fictional "biochemical imbalance and

> (c)no psychiatric drug has ever constantly outperformed a placebo in clinical trials...to cure a malady one has to locate it."(Tribune Review, May 16, 2017)

According to the <u>"Physician's Desk Reference 1996"</u> that include candid information by the drug companies (to avoid law suits), the following side effect are listed (among others):

nervousness, insomnia, dyskinesia, Tourette syndrome, toxic psychosis

The list is followed by the following statement:

"Long term effect of Ritalin in children have not been well established."

(Cited in the New American, s. a.)

The Medicines and Healthcare Products Regulatory Agency (MHRA) (FDA's British counterpart) concluded that SSRIs should not be used (except Prozac) to treat adolescents with major depressive disorder. (AMA-journal of Ethics, June 2012)

The International Narcotic Control Board (of which America is a member) informed that <u>90 % of the drug was produced and consumed in the US.</u> (s. United Nations's warning in chapter19)

There were law-suits filed in connection with Ritalin. In Texas, a school sued parents who refused to have their child treated with Ritalin. The judge decided that if the parents could find a psychiatrist who agreed with them they could refuse treatment. (s. Chapter 19)

In Georgia parents sued school officials and doctors because they had not been advised of Ritalin's severe side effects. (<u>www.edforce.house.gov/hearings/106th/oi/ritalin92900</u>)

There is also a monetary aspect that plays into the Ritalin situation. The Supplemental Security Income (SSI) provides money to low-income parents whose children are diagnosed as having ADHD-which the government accepts as learning disability, and many dollars in special education grant money are given to schools.

Psychiatrist <u>Stanley Greenspan</u> writes in his book "Overcoming ADHD (2009) that difficulties with ADD and ADHD can be overcome with other means which he points out in detail in his book. Pills should be the last resort. "It's not about sitting still". "We have to find the underlying causes." He feels that "many children on medication experience a restriction in their emotional range." (p.12).

And Dr. <u>Robert S. Mendelsohn</u>, a pediatrician who wrote "How to Raise a Healthy Child…In Spite of Your Doctor" (1984) wrote: "If your child's teacher, school principal, counselor or pediatrician attempts to pressure you into accepting chemical treatment for his behavior pattern, reject the advice out of hand. There is no benefit for your child that justifies the risks nor can they be justified in order to spare his teacher the annoyance of having him talk out of turn or squirm in his seat" (Cited in The New American, s.a.)

15. Comments and criticism regarding ADHD and its treatment

<u>Rick Mayes</u>, a public policy analyst, a former NIMH employee and postdoctoral fellow (I assume in public policy) has written a book about this subject with his two co-authors, Catherine Bagwell, child psychologist and Jennifer Erkulwater, political scientist, under the title <u>"Medicating children – ADHD and Pediatric Mental Health." (2009)</u> Despite a wealth of cited sources that are critical of the ADHD diagnosis and treatment, there are statements in the book that cannot be proven, e.g. he claims that there has been "a sizable growth in knowledge about ADHD" (p.2), but writes a few pages later "there is no medical (blood, urine, radiological) test to verify an ADHD diagnosis." (p.5)

He cites three reasons that explain the surge in ADHD diagnoses and stimulant use.(p.3) (I cite Mayes verbally):

1.) "In 1990, a Supreme Court ruling led to a modification of the Supplemental Security Income (SSI) program which provides financial assistance for individuals with disabilities –to include low income-children diagnosed with mental disorders such as ADHD. Congress later rescinded this expansion, but before that the rate of children enrolled in the program increased almost threefold.

2.) Due to large lobbying pressure from parents of children with ADHD (according to a report from the United Nations, these parent groups were paid by the drug companies, s. following article "The United Nations"), Congress in 1991 urged the Department of Education to clarify that ADHD was a protected disability under the Individuals with Disabilities Education Act (IDEA). As a result, more children diagnosed with the disorder became eligible for special accommodations... <u>low income children with ADHD could receive cash assistance for their families from SSR.</u>

3.) Beginning in the early 1990, policy makers expanded tremendously the number of individuals, especially children, eligible for Medicaid. As a result, between 1988 and 1993, the total number of children receiving Medicaid services grew by 53%. [This] "fueled massive increases in Medicaid spending on psychotropic drugs in general –from \$0.6 billion in 1991 to \$6.7 billion in 2001 and particularly on stimulants...spending per child on stimulants grew almost ninefold..." (p.3)

The authors explain the two views on mental disorders, the

    a) <u>Biological view</u> –"which stresses the neurosciences, brain chemistry and psychotropic medication " (which is ironic because <u>no</u> chemical in the brain has been found by scientists to cause mental disorders) and

    b) <u>Psychodynamic or psychosocial view</u> - ..."which sees mental disorders as largely influenced by individuals' personalities,...social problems and personal stress." (p.3, 4)

The authors point to the negative role the pharmaceutical companies play in this situation:

> "<u>The DSM-III</u> provided much more specific diagnoses for drug companies to target their products <u>which...has led to a disconcerting level of financial interconnectedness among clinical researchers, physicians and the pharmaceutical industry.</u> For example, 13 of the 21 individuals who created the most recent version of the DSM criteria for ADHD had financial ties to the pharmaceutical companies that market stimulants." (p. 7)

They cite Steven Hyman, provost of Harvard University and former director of the National Institute of Mental Health "...we don't connect the wires in our own lives about how money is affecting our profession."(of psychiatrists) (p.7)

Amazingly, the authors come to the conclusion (remember, none of them is a psychiatrist or trained in natural science): "The reality is that there is an abundance of research finding from the past 3 decades that strongly suggests that ADHD is a real disorder and that stimulants are a generally safe and effective treatment for it when used properly." (p.11) Instead of examining the huge controversy and the stated danger and therefor warning of stimulants by the FDA, the authors only cite one article. They use nebulous language: "most children are on something of a continuum in terms of their vulnerability (as is now the dominant conceptualization of autism spectrum disorders." (p.11) (What are they saying?)

They state: "Arguably the most important thing for many clinicians and parents regarding an ADHD diagnosis that it provides the basis for financial reimbursement by health insurance companies..." (p.12)

They point out that

They write that mood and anxiety disorders and many other mental disorders are connected to ADHD (which opens a wide field of treatment possibilities) and they are not critical of the influence of the pharmaceutical industry. (p.18)

Talking about medication for ADHD, (Ritalin, Dexedrine, Adderall and Concerta) the authors state "In most cases, the side effects are mild." (p.34) (they should have cited the FDA's warning about stimulants, including warnings about suicide). They do admit, however:" there has been some concern about their cardiovascular safety."(p.34) Talking about Adderall XR (extended release) "when children have underlying heart anomalies (often silent):

> According to the FDA there are 12 known cases of sudden death...and in Canada the sale of Adderall XR has been suspended. "[This] did not result in suspension of Adderall XR sales in the United States...it was concluded that the rate of sudden deaths ...was not significantly higher than would be expected without treatment." (p. 34)

The authors admit that "not all children who take stimulant medication demonstrate significant improvement in their symptoms, perhaps 10%-20% do not "(p.35)) They further describe psychosocial treatment (like parent management) and a combination of medical and psychosocial treatment. They claim that "In terms of treatment with medication in the MTA (Multimodal treatment study of children with ADHD) ...By the end of the study 73% were successfully maintained on methylphenidate[Ritalin]..." (p.37) They continue: "This MTA study ...is arguably the most thorough and detailed study of treatment effectiveness, not only for ADHD, but for any psychiatric disorder in childhood...use of higher doses to maximize effectiveness and minimize side effects) (this makes no sense at all)...may be responsible for the improvement with MTA protocols over community care" (p.38). They conclude "combined medication and psychosocial treatment yielded no substantial improvement over medication alone." (p.42)

I googled MTA (which was sponsored by the National Institute for Mental Health (NIMH)) and found many websites praising this study, among them government related ones. A parent seeking information could probably easily be convinced that medical treatment of ADHD is the best method to deal with this problem. However, when you dig a little deeper, you find an article by Peter Breggin, the "conscience of psychiatry" in which he conducts a critical examination of this study. He found several flaws:

- (I) The MTA was not a placebo-controlled, double blind-clinical trial. (There was no placebo control group and no no treatment control group)
- The researchers relied on parents' and teachers' evaluations who knew whether the children were taken the medication. ("open label") "The sponsors and all the principal investigators were staunch advocates of medication."
- (2) The MAT used one group of "blind raters" who observed the students only in the classroom. <u>They found no difference in the treatment groups</u>, i.e.

1.) the group who only took medication
2.) the group that was treated with a combination of medicine and behavioral therapy
3.) the group that received behavioral therapy alone and
4.) the group that received routine community treatment.(?)

This was an essential finding, but "was not considered in the study conclusion."

- (III) There was no control group of untreated children. (no placebo)
- (IV) Thirty- two percent of the Medication Management Group was already on medication for ADHD at the start of the study.
- (V) The Medication Management was highly selective... and probably not typical for children seeking services for ADHD.

Originally there were 4,541 children, of those only 579 were chosen for the study. (Breggin feels that that does not represent a community of children routinely treated for "ADHD" and that many of them already took stimulant medication.

- (VI) The Medication Management group was… small:

Of the 579 who entered the clinical trials, only 144 received the medication alone. Thirteen dropped out before starting, eight more dropped out during the study, so only 123 (2.7 percent) remained in the medication management group.

- (VII) The children did not rate themselves improved (as doing better on the drugs than on any other treatment.) "This result supports the use of safer non-drug treatment."
- (VIII) Most of the subjects were boys. (Breggin interpretes this that "stimulants are used to suppress the relatively higher activity rates of normal boys compared to girls.")
- (IX) Drug treatment continued for fourteen months; behavioral treatments were stopped earlier. Breggin states that this "gives the drug treatment an unfair advantage."
- (X) The behavioral treatments were flawed. ("They showed no advantage to drugs.")
- (XI) Most children suffered from adverse drug reactions. (ADRs)
- (XII) There were no trained observers for ADRs.

Parents and teachers were the observers. "There was no apparent training for this process…parents and teachers were reassured …that the drug was safe and that the ARDs were not serious…Furthermore, many ADRs—such as behavioral suppression, loss of spontaneity, apathy, and increased obsessive behavior – are mistakenly interpreted as improvements by parents and teachers."

Breggin also criticizes that the children were not asked how the drugs made them feel. He writes:

"The study failed to carry out an objective evaluation of long-term adverse effects that have already been demonstrated in short-term studies. For example, the study should have gathered data on physical parameters such as height and weight (growth), blood pressure, cardiac status, and abnormal movements, as well as on psychological parameters…it is obvious that the investigators did not intend to evaluate the …most important issue surrounding the long-term use – the risks they pose to children."

- (XIII) There was no improvement in academic performance.
- (XIV) There was very little effects on social skills.
- (XV) All the principal investigators were well-known drug advocates. "They touted the positive results of the study even before it was completed or published." One of the investigators was Lawrence Greenhill of the New York State Psychiatric Institute and Columbia University. Their website "originally listed the funding of its researchers. (NYSPI Sponsored Research (1998). Greenhill had research funds or other financial support from six drug companies: Richwood, Brystol-Myers, Solvay, Wyeth-Ayerst, Glaxo and Eli Lilly."
- The parents and teachers were exposed to pro drug propaganda in the material that was given to them before the study. "Parents were not given the opportunity for informed consent for the risks posed to their children by the drugs."

(CiteSeerX (https://citeseerx.ist.psu.edu> document A Critical   Analysis of the NIMH Multimodal Treatment Study for Attention- Deficit/Hyperactivity Disorder. (The MTA Study)

Other authors are also very critical of the ADHD diagnoses and their chemical treatment.

One of them is the psychologist John Rosemond, author of the book (together with pediatrician Bose Ravenel) "The Diseasing of America's Children". He claims that any supposed scientific explanation does not really hold water. He writes: [it is an]

> "effort by the unholy alliance of psychology, psychiatry, pediatric neurology and big pharma to proliferate the spurious diagnosis."
> (Tribune Review, Nov. 1, 2016)

In another article Rosemond writes:

> "No one has proven the reality of ADHD. oppositional defiance disorder or bipolar disorder in childhood. They are constructs... Drugs to "treat" childhood behavior disorders are based on theories that no researcher has ever established as true. That is why pharmaceuticals do not reliably outperform placebos in clinical trials."

He quotes Harvard psychologist Jerome Kagan as saying that ADHD is "an invention."(Tribune Review , April 11, 2017) In another article Rosemond looks at the prescriptions given to children diagnosed with ADHD, especially methylphenidates (MPH) like Ritalin or Concerta. He says that they affect brain function. They are stimulants, classified by the Drug Enforcement Administration (DEA) as Schedule 2 narcotics, the same classification given to cocaine, morphine and amphetamines. He continues: " A 2019 study published online in Neuroradiology found that

> after 16 weeks of MPH "treatment" the brains of preteen boys (10-12) showed statistically significant cognitive aging as determined by measures of FA (?)...A placebo group of boys showed no cognitive aging...In other words, the damage to the brain... done by the MPH was exclusive to the preteen group, compromised of kids whose brains are still in development...There are [potentially] very serious permanent dangers to their children...Bear in mind that the study found the cognitive aging effect of MPH to be significant only after 16 weeks of administration. Most of the ADHD-diagnosed kids I run across have been taken MPH for years...Scary is a word that pops to mind. So does immoral." (Tribune Revue, Sept.1, 2019)

I finally want to point out an article written by an Education reporter for the <u>Eagle Forum</u> Education & Legal Defense Fund of July 1996.
The reporter points out the following:

> " In 1991 the U.S. Department of Education formally recognized ADHD as a handicap under the Individuals with Disabilities Education Act and section 504 of the 1973 Rehabilitation Act<u>." All state education officers had to ensure that local school districts establish procedures to screen and identify ADHD children and give them special educational and psychological services."</u>

He writes "generous funding suddenly began to flow."

 <u>Peter Breggin</u> recommends a re-evaluation when your child takes medication for ADHD. He has written several books about the subject and says the following (in his book "Your drug may be your problem" (1999)): "When children are taken off ADHD-drugs you have to be very careful and slow and be guided by an expert and

you have to watch out for withdrawal symptoms." (p.174). You should find out if the child has been put on drugs because of school problems or home problems. If you are confused or inconsistent as a parent you might see that this is the main cause of your child's problems. When you medicate your child, you avoid self examination as a parent. He writes: "for parents every child is a new challenge. Some traits like high energy and independence may be testing your parental skills." (p.177) He feels that many parents keep their children on drugs or even use them as kind of babysitters. He calls this "parent attention deficit disorder" (p.177). To take your child off drugs might lead to the most important decision in your life – to spend more time with your child." (p.178) He feels that particularly boys, need a strong father who teaches discipline and respectful behavior. But, he cautions, the father should not act as a pal and he should not avoid disciplinary actions, because this encourages the child to take advantage of mother or other caregivers. (p.178). He encourages play-acting with toy animals, e.g. to reveal how the child feels during withdrawal.

Focusing on school problems, Breggin points out that originally children were prescribed stimulants to help with discipline problems, but that they now were prescribed for improved academic performance. He emphasizes that there is no proof for this, on the contrary: that these medications "are more likely to impair mental functioning." (p. 179) He also suggests that you ask the teacher's help to increase your child's attention in class, like individualized instruction. (Some children are highly intelligent, "get it" the first time and get bored when the teacher keeps repeating a concept to the slower students.) He continues: "Some teacher give better grades to children on drugs because the drugs make them more conforming. But better grades are not worth the price of drug-induced conformity." He says: "Stop struggling with your child about homework and focus on enjoying parenthood... In our opinion, nothing is more important than the quality of your personal relationship with your child. Don't stress out about grades: As your child grows up, he or she will have multiple opportunities to develop an interest in school and education. So, whereas future opportunities for school abound, your child will never be able to get a new brain unaffected by drugs." (p.180, 181)

Breggin gives the following advice when the school insists to put your child on drugs:

- Work closely with school

- Spend time in the classroom and observe your child
- Consult an independent counselor or switch schools
- Tell the teacher: "I know that Ritalin has a good chance of making my child more compliant in class, but that's just not the kind of improvement I want for my child. I do not beat my child if he suffers a setback in class, and I refuse to drug my child for the same purpose."(p. 182)

Psychiatrist <u>Stanley Greenspan</u> (in his book <u>"Overcoming ADHD</u> " (2009)) has similar thoughts. He asks if children and adults with an ADHD diagnosis can overcome their difficulties without pills. And he answer this question with an absolute yes for the "vast majority". (p.2) He feels that there are "many different roads that lead to the symptoms". (p.2). For example, he feels that some children are highly sensitive to sights, sounds and other sensations and are therefore easily distracted, others crave those and are "constantly on the move... others withdraw into their imagination, some have difficulty with visualizing." (p. 2,3) He feels that "treatments only focus on reducing the outward signs of the disorder." (p.3) "Some children focus on TV and find it hard to shift their attention to people even if their mothers or fathers are calling them." He says that there are many successful people who would have gotten the label of ADHD. Greenspan always does a six to 12 month trial before he considers medication. He says that there are many children who don't require medication. If he feels that medication is necessary "it is likely to be a lesser dose and of lesser duration". He feels "that many children (on these drugs) experience a constriction in their emotional range ... Their creativity or sense of humor may not be as great" (p.12) Like Breggin, he feels that family dynamics play an important part in this diagnosis, that sometimes prescribing a pill is the easy way out and that much can be done to improve this condition with other means than a pill.

In regard to the dangers pointed out above, the **United Nations** released in 1995 the following statement:

> **the <u>United Nation</u>, in its annual report, the UN's International Narcotics Control Board, issued a warning about <u>Ritalin</u> (Methylphenidate) under the title "Dramatic Increase in Methylphenidate Consumption in US: Marketing Methods**

Questioned". The report states that the drug was classified as a
schedule II drug as having high abuse potential. The international
Narcotics Control Board has observed a world use of
Methylphenidate rose from 3 tonnes in 1990 to more than 8.5
tonnes in 1994, and continued to rise. The United States accounts
for about 90 percent of total world manufacture and consumption.
The …sharp increase is due to its controversially extensive use in
the treatment of ADD (now called ADHD) in children. The INCB
shares its concern with the US Drug Enforcement Agency (DEA) The
danger the Board sees is overpresciption. Also, the duration of
treatment is restricted in many countries to three years, it tends to
be much longer in the US… many children remain on it into
adolescence, even adulthood although there are no tests that
examine the side effects of such long-term treatment.
There is an increase of abuse of Ritalin with serious damage to
health like addiction and stimulant –abuse symptoms.
"The INCB is also concerned that the use of Ritalin is being actively
promoted by an influential parent association which has received
significant contribution from the "the US manufacturer of the drug.
"This association has petitioned the DEA to ease the control …"
"At the present, the unprecedented high level of ADD [ADHD] in
children, the very widespread prescription of Ritalin and the
growing abuse and black market appear to be limited to the United
States" The board sees a danger that these problems will take hold
in other countries and states that some of the parent groups
indicated that they will promote the use in other countries.
"The Board is therefore requesting all governments to exercise
utmost vigilance to prevent the overdiagnosing of ADD and any
medically-unjustified treatment with Methylphenidate and other
stimulants. It has also requested the World Health Organization
(WHO) to investigate this matter and to provide expertise to
national public health authorities."

The report adds the following:

"…Concern has been raised that doctors are resorting to
Methylphenidate as an "easy" solution for behavioral problems

which may have complex causes. Critics warn that parents' and teachers' assessments of what constitutes "inattention" and "impulsivity" are highly subjective and that doctors'prescribing practices for Methylphenidate are far from uniform."
(Source : QWQED-FRONTLINE)

There is some hope that schoolboards take a more critical view in regard to drug treatment. There is an article published by the NLM (National Library of Medicine) which is part of the NIH.(with a disclaimer) of wjm(western journal of medicine) in February 2000); 172(2): 80-81, (PMCID: PMC1070779, PMID: 18751234) with   the title:
<u>US board of education advises against drugs for behavioral problems,</u>
written by Fred Charatan. I quote:

"A US board of education has passed a resolution urging teachers to use discipline and instruction to overcome problem behavior in the classroom, rather than encouraging parents to seek drug treatment for their children.
The resolution passed by Colorado Board of Education carries no legal weight but sounds a warning on the growing use of drugs such as Ritalin… to deal with disruptive behavior in schools. Board members supporting the resolution believed that
<u>many violent crimes committed by school students are committed by young people taking psychotropic drugs</u>. In the massacre last spring at Columbine High School in Lillleton, Colorado, one of the teenage shooters, Eric Harris, had been taking the antidepressant Luvox…

The board's action, believed to be the first in the United States, is sure to intensify the debate over the use of psychotropic drugs in conditions such as attention deficit hyperactivity disorder. An estimated 2.5 million children in the United States are now taking drugs for this type of problem.
Peter Breggin…believes that doctors are overprescribing psychotropic drugs. 'It's a tremendous mistake to subdue the behavior of children instead of tending to their needs.' He is

99

convinced that <u>there is a direct link between the drugs and violent acts.</u>"

16. ADHD medications' impact on learning

Similar to the MAT-study that I wrote about in chapter 15, the Florida International University has conducted a study to determine if stimulants or other psychotropic medication had an impact on learning. The study was funded by the National Institute on Mental Health. (NIMH). The researchers (the researcher responsible for this study was a distinguished professor of psychology at FIU, William E. Pelham jr.) found that <u>medication alone had no impact on learning</u>. (To read the study go to <u>https://news.fiu.edu>long thought to be the key to a ...</u>)
The article describing the study was written on May 23, 2022 by Rosanna Castro, a professional and member of the research team. She writes:

> "For decades, most physicians, parents and teachers have believed that stimulant medication helps children with ADHD learn. However, in the first study of its kind, researchers at the Center for Children and Families at FIU found that <u>medication has no detectable impact on how much children with ADHD learn in the classroom</u>...most physicians believe that medication will result in better academic achievement...Physicians and educators have held the belief that medication helps children with ADHD learn, because they complete more seatwork and spend more time on-task when medicated", said William E. Pelham jr., senior author of the study and director of the Center for children and families.)

He wrote:

> "Unfortunately we found <u>that medication had no impact on learning of actual curriculum content.</u> Contrary to expectation, research found that children learned the same amount of science, social studies and vocabulary content whether they were taking the medication or the placebo. While medication did not improve learning, [it] helped children complete more seat-work and improve their classroom behavior... When taking medication, children completed 37 percent more arithmetic problems per minute and committed 53 percent fewer classroom rules violations per hour....Additionally...researchers found that medication slightly

helped to improve test scores when medication is taken on the day of the test, but not enough to boost most children's grades. For example, medication helped children increase an average 1.7 percentage points out of 100 on science and social studies tests."

The authors found through research that behavior therapy – when used first – is less expensive and more effective as a first line treatment. They state: "Medicating our children doesn't solve the problem – it only takes the symptoms temporarily … families should …add medication only when needed."

17. Side effects of best-known psychotropic drugs listed by experts

The English psychiatrist <u>Joanna Moncrieff</u> is very critical of psychiatric drugs. In her book "<u>A straight talking introduction to psychiatric drugs</u>"(2020), she writes that laboratory experiments showed that stimulants like Ritalin improved people's performance in the short term, but impair these at higher doses. (p.112) She also cites children's descriptions of their feelings after taking stimulants:" '[It] numbed me'; 'It makes me sad'; 'It takes over of me'; 'Don't feel like myself'. (p.113) The author points out that "controlled studies do not show evidence of beneficial effects on school achievement in children" (p.114) She also points out that

> "many of the studies in children and adults have been conducted by...researchers at Harvard University who were revealed to have <u>received millions of dollars from the pharmaceutical industry."</u>

(source cited on p.114)

Moncrieff is very concerned about the harmful effects of stimulants (p.116-119) such as

- The suppression of growth (up to 2.6 cm)
- A possible delay in puberty (both probably due to hormonal influence)
- Heart problems, namely an increase in heart rate and blood pressure that can result in deaths (when taking higher doses.)
- The development of Parkinson's disease. (It is seven times higher in people who used stimulants)
- The development of mental disorders like psychosis, depression, anxiety, agitation, insomnia, abnormal movements like twitches and tics. (In 8- 9% of children. (Source cited on p.118)
- Tolerance to the drug and therefor the danger of addiction
- Withdrawal symptoms (fatigue and depression)
- <u>The rebound effect, i.e. the reappearance and possible increase in the symptoms that the drug is supposed to eliminate.</u> ("often interpreted as re-emergence of the underlying symptoms and taken as confirmation that continued treatment is necessary." (p. 119)

Moncrieff sees also a danger because it makes the child believe to have a disease that can't be helped and that a diagnosis might keep a child from trying to work on his problems and to learn to master them.

Peter Breggin in his book "Talking back to Ritalin" (1998) lists a group of drugs that are used to treat ADHD. These are Ritalin, Dexedrine, Dextrostat, Adderall, Desoxyn, Gradumet and Cylert. He says (Appendix A, p.357,358)

> " Except for Cylert, all of these drugs have nearly identical effects and side effects…"

- Ritalin and amphetamine have almost identical effects on the brain, mind and behavior including the production of drug-induced behavioral disorders, psychosis, mania, drug abuse and addiction.
- Ritalin and amphetamine frequently cause the very same problems they are supposed to treat-inattention, hyperactivity and impulsivity.
- A large percentage of children become robotic, lethargic, depressed, or withdrawn (from the use of stimulants.)
- Ritalin can cause permanent neurological tics including Tourette's syndrome.
- Ritalin can retard growth in children by disrupting the cycles of growth hormone released by the pituitary gland.
- The recent findings that Ritalin can cause cancer in some animals was not taken seriously enough by the drug company or the FDA.

Breggin points out the danger of withdrawal including depression and suicide. He states that depression might lead to a new cycle of prescriptions, that the drug might also become a gateway to other addictions, that the U.S. uses 90% of the world's Ritalin, that the drug has no positive effect on the child's psychology or academic performance or that there is no evidence that ADHD is a genuine disorder.(p. 358, 359) He also writes that

> "The U.S. Department of Education and the National Institute of Mental Health (NIMH) push Ritalin…vigorously." (p.360)

Breggin writes that it was an Eli Lilli researcher, D. T. Wong, who published the first article about this medication in 1974. He writes that

and that this company began marketing this drug by 1988. He lists four drugs that
are Selective Serotonin Reuptake inhibitors (in 1994):

           Zoloft (Sertraline)
           Paxil   (Paroxetine)
           Luvox (Fluvoxamine)
and   Serzone (Nefazadone)

Breggin warns that once a drug is approved for marketing by the FDA, there are
no government controls for what it can prescribed for. ("off label") He lists the
problems that are treated with SSRSs :

- Winter Blues
- Obesity
- Anorexia
- Bulimia
- Phobias
- Anxiety
- Panic disorder
- Chronic Fatigue Symptom
- Premenstrual Syndrome
- Postpartum Depression
- Drug and Alcohol Addiction
- Migraine Headaches
- Arthritis
- Body Dysmorphic Disorder (imagined unattractiveness of self)
- Behavioral and emotional disorders in children and adolescents

The author writes that soon "the darker side" of the drug appeared: the
emotional damage or even death caused by the drug.
The FDA held hearings on this issue in 1991. In 1992 Eli Lilly reported to the
Security and Exchange Commission: "170 actions to recover damages as result of
ingestion of Prozac"

He points out that "law-suits were brought for alleged negligence in prescribing drugs or in criminal courts as defense for having committed crimes "and that there is a Prozac survivor group."

The article "Antidepressants" in Wikipedia (accessed April 27, 2024) shows 297 scientific sources and reveals the following: they are the most commonly prescribed medication in America. They are used for many diseases, even purely physical ones. Their side effects are: increased suicidal thinking and actions in children, adolescents and young adults. A discontinuation syndrome may occur after stopping which resembles depression. Sexual dysfunction may be permanent. Research regarding effectiveness is controversial… evidence of benefits in children and adolescents is…inconclusive. "Other researchers… concluded that antidepressants ultimately do more harm than good, indicating that they cause permanent neuronal damage, apoptosis (natural death of cells) and disrupt numerous adaptive processes regulated by Serotonin". "Despite its longstanding prominence in pharmaceutical advertising the myth that low serotonin levels cause depression is not supported by scientific evidence. "

"Misreporting of clinical trial outcomes and of serious side effects such as suicide, is common."

One adverse side effect is serotonin toxicity which is an excess of serotonin that can cause mania, restlessness, agitation, emotional lability, insomnia, confusion. SSRIs can cause suicidal thinking, heart problems, birth defects, mania, sexual dysfunction, emotional blunting, gaining or losing weight, a reduction in bone density in the lumbar spine, an increased risk of death (+33 %) and cardiovascular complications. The above mentioned English psychiatrist Joanna Moncrieff and colleagues showed that the serotonin theory of depression was not supported by evidence.

(Again, this Wikipedia article cites 297 scientific sources that can all be easily accessed)

Psychologist Bruce Levine in his book "A Profession without Reason" (2022) is also very critical of the pharmaceutical industry. He writes about psychiatrist and former NIHM director Thomas Insel: "He had rejected the validity of psychiatry's DSM…and he had challenged the idea that all individuals with serious mental illness …need to remain on medications long term and…had acknowledged psychiatry's abysmal treatment outcomes." (p. 26) He had found that treatment of mental illness had –from 1992 to 2002- increased from 20% to 33%, but that the results had not changed for the same time period. Levine could only affirm Insel's statement. He describes the <u>poor outcome despite increased treatment.</u> He writes:

> "Between 1988 and 2008, the rate of antidepressant use in the United States increased nearly 400 percent, yet outcomes only have worsened." (p. 27)

He states that the CDC (Centers for Disease Control) reported in 2020 that from 1999 to 2018 the suicide rate increased 35% and that the mental illness disability was 1 in every 184 Americans in 1987, but it more than doubled to 1 in every 76 Americans in 2007 and he quotes the World Health Organization (WHO) who reported in 2020 "There is 10-25 year life expectancy reduction in patients with severe mental disorders…Mortality rate among people with schizophrenia is 2 to 2.5 higher than the general population" (p.27)

Levine reports about an incident that *60 Minutes* reporter Katie Couric (Sept. 30, 2007) "What killed <u>Rebeccah Riley?</u>" related. Rebecca died as a 4 year- old in 2006. When Rebecca was 28 months old, her mother complained about her being hyper and having insomnia and asked a psychiatrist for help. The psychiatrist diagnosed ADHD and put her on <u>Clonidine,</u> a hypertensive medication and sedative. That medication had also been prescribed to Rebecca's older brother and sister. When Rebecca was three the doctor diagnosed also bipolar disorder and prescribed, in addition, the antipsychotic <u>Seroquel</u> and the anticonvulsant <u>Depacote</u>. The parents had added two cough medications and the little girl died at four years old. Her parents sedated the children to make them easier to control and they got a psychiatric diagnosis to be able to get disability payments. The parents were charged with murder and convicted, but the psychiatrist did not only remain free, but also continues to practice. (p. 48)

Levine also writes that the chemical imbalance theory has been disproved since 1990. Professor Elliot Walenstein showed that it is just as likely for people with normal serotonin levels to feel depressed as it is for people with abnormally low   serotonin levels. The APA informed the general public in 2000 in that regard by stating:" The exact causes of mental disorders are unknown, but an explosive growth of research has brought us closer to the answers." (p.89). (s. Mayes, Rick et al.) (The second part of the sentence is nebulous and might lead the trusting patient to believe that science is close to an answer which it is not.) Levine feels that the first part of this statement) is not clear and loud enough. He writes:

> "A 2006 survey reveals that 80 percent of Americans believed that depression is caused by a chemical imbalance…Prior to the public's acceptance of the chemical imbalance cause of depression, many people were reluctant to take antidepressants –or to give them to their children. "(p. 89, 90)

My special concern is about <u>coerced antipsychotic medication</u>. I am thinking about children, adolescents and adults like prisoners who are forced to take medication, usually through the legal system. (s. chapter 22 about children in foster care.) Are the judges even familiar with the problems that the DSM presents? Or with the side effects of the medication prescribed? That many of the unwanted behaviors like aggression are the result of taking these medications? It breaks my heart to read that juveniles are punished severely for behaviors that are the results of drugs that they were often forced to take? Levine writes: "…there is a great deal of research that challenges the value of these medications for long –term use." (p.130) Levine lists several studies , some of them conducted by WHO that showed that patients with mental illness off medication recovered at a higher rate than those that were maintained on drugs. (p.130/131) He in particular cites a study by psychiatrist Courtenay Harding in 1985. She found that the "common factor shared by the best- outcome group was that they had all successfully weaned themselves from antipsychotic drugs." (p.131)

He also mentions researcher Martin Harrow, who had found in an NIMH-funded study that after 15 years, patients who were diagnosed with schizophrenia, 40 percent of those who had stopped medication were judged to be in recovery compared to only 5 percent who had remained on antipsychotic drugs. Levine continues:

> "Those off medication fared better on every measure (Including the presence of psychotic symptoms, relapse rate, anxiety level, cognitive functioning and employment" (p 131, 132)

Harrow concluded: "The …data raise questions about prolonged treatment of schizophrenia with antipsychotic medications." (p.132) In 2013 researcher Lex Wunderink published a study that showed that after seven years 40 percent of patients who had discontinued their medication had recovered versus 18 percent who had remained on them". (p.132)

18. Patient groups

Ray Moynihan and Alan Cassels point out some interesting facts about ADHD in their book "Selling Sickness". (2005) They identify the "influential parent association" that I wrote about before and that is mentioned in the cited report of the United Nations as CHADD (Children and Adults with Attention-Deficit /Hyperactivity Disorder.) At the time their book was published, CHADD had fifteen thousand members and two hundred affiliates. (p.61). They state that it is mostly white affluent neighborhoods that show an ADD[H] epidemic. 20 percent of young white boys are now taking "speed-like stimulants for their ADD."(p.62) In the decade from 1990 the production of the drug rose almost 800 percent. By 2000, with under 5 percent of the world's population, Americans were consuming 800 percent.
Compared to this in Europe, 5% of children and adolescents are taking these drugs.(https://www.cdc.gov>ncbadd>adhd>data)

The authors point out that partnering with patient groups has become an important marketing tool. (p. 62) Many health charities and patient groups accept now support from drug or device manufacturers. (p.62) CHADD receives almost $700,000 annually. (In 2013 one million a year, according to the New York Times, Dec. 14, 2013) (I could not access a more recent number).The authors admit that there are children who have severe symptoms of the disease who will be helped with medical intervention but because of the "scientific uncertainty" other influences like environment etc. should be considered and changed to help the child.(s. Dr. Robert Mendelson, Dr. Peter Breggin) They point out that "there is no reliable test for it, and no strong evidence that it is biologically determined."(p.64) Even, they write, the NIH is admitting this. The authors continue:
> "It is obvious that viewing ADD as a biochemical disorder greatly
> benefits the companies selling chemicals that purport to fix it.
> [CHADD also "promotes the condition as a …neurobiological
> disorder. "(p. 64)]

The authors mention a drug company, Shire, that sells more than $520 million dollars of Adderall every year" (p.65) A slide from this company showed a pyramid indicating the people it was trying to influence. In the top part were the "medical decision makers that the company tried to influence through sponsored education efforts." (p.65), at the bottom the patients it was trying to influence through "Medical Societies" and "Medical Advocacy Groups." (p.66) The authors continue about CHADD: " it is one of the highest profile patient advocacy group in the U.S. It offers CHADD certified training and support to other parents. CHADD admits some scientific uncertainty but claims that ADD "has a very strong neurological basis." CHADD claims that 'medication is the most effective foundation for treatment.' (p.66). The authors point out that <u>the group accepted three quarters of a million dollars in the early 1990 from Ciba-Geigy, then makers of Ritalin.</u> The U.S. government DEA (Drug Enforcement Agency) was alarmed about the spiraling use of Ritalin and other ADD drugs and warned: "The relationship between Ciba-Geigy and CHADD raises serious concerns about CHADD's motive in proselytizing the use of Ritalin" (source cited on p. 67) The authors bemoan the fact <u>that the public is often unaware of the connection between business and disease.</u> (They also point out that the industry found a new market (adult ADHD) and say ironically :" the lifespan of an adult's potential drug-taking is much, much longer."(p. 68))

Another important patient group is <u>NAMI (</u>National Alliance for the Mentally Ill), according to Bruce Levine, <u>"the recipient of Eli Lilly funding."</u> The New York Times reported: "...according to investigators in [Senator]...Grassley's office and documents obtained by the New York Times, drug makers from 2006 to 2008 contributed nearly $23 million to the Alliance." (cited from "Drug makers are advocacy groups Biggest Donors", by Gardiner Harris, N.Y.Times, Oct.21.2009.)

The authors describe further the "branding of a condition". They cite the marketing professional Vince Parry. "Parry says drug companies will often bring the key players together-the thought leaders, the local physicians and the patient groups- to help define, refine and brand new conditions." For him, an aim is "elevating the importance of an unknown condition." (p.70). The authors state that men like Parry "fundamentally change the way we think our bodies, our health, and the conditions we supposedly suffer." (p. 71) They cite a sociology professor who saw the problem of "medicalizing human problems:"(p. 76) "The increasing tendency to define unpleasant human feelings and troublesome behavior as a 'disease' to be corrected with drugs."(p.76) He felt that that approach keeps people from seeking real solutions to their problems and "depoliticize [s]'social problems".(p.76) They cite the pediatrician Dr. Lawrence

Diller who said "I began to wonder if boyhood …had become a disease." (p.76)
Diller claims that a key factor is very important.: "a change to federal disability
laws…which meant that if a child had a diagnosis of ADD, it could lead to special
educational services for that child at school."(p. 77)
Also by widening the definition of ADD like "<u>often does not seem to listen</u>" the
pool of students being diagnosed becomes larger and larger. (50 percent more in
1987 than in1980) The authors point out that amphetamines also have an effect
on normal children and cite a scientist who says "Football players and race horses
have known that for a longtime" (cited on p.79). They state that
<u>sales for</u> <u>stimulants have grown immensely, especially for children under five</u>.
They also mention that the clinical trials have been short and "poorly run." They
suggest that the ADD "epidemic" is not due to faulty biochemistry but rather to a
much more complex mix of many factors –including the well-funded "condition
branding" designed by Vince Parry and his colleagues in Manhattan. (p. 80)

In his book "<u>Childhood under Siege – how Big Business Targets Children</u>"
(2011) <u>Joel Bakan</u>, professor of law at the University of British Columbia, Canada,
takes a closer look at the medicalization of our children. He points out that in the

DSM-1 (1952) there was no reference to childhood disorders
DSM-2 (1968) there were 2 pages)
DSM-3 (1980) there were 65 pages identifying childhood disorders, 5 pages alone
            devoted to ADD) (p.73)

He points out that between 1980 and 1990 the diagnosis of ADD and ADHD rose
from 400,000 to 900,000, the treatment with drugs from 28 % to 86%. (p.73) He
writes that drugs became the first line treatment for kids' emotional and
behavioral problems:

> "Its many pages of …presumptively biological disorders gave
> pharmaceutical companies the targets they needed to develop and
> market new drugs, and psychiatrists the reason …to prescribe them."
> (p.73)
> "DSM-V (sic) scheduled for release in 2013, could push psychiatry
> even deeper into the arms of the pharmaceutical industry by

including...sub-threshold (such as *mild depression*) and premorbid (such as *prepsychotic*) categories." (p.83)

Like others here mentioned, he writes that the Bay-Dole act of 1980 allowed scientist and institutions ownership of their discoveries although these were funded by the taxpayer. This allowed them to become marketable, i.e. they could be sold to corporations.

"Soon after...pharmaceutical money poured into medical research" (p.74), companies became increasingly involved in the conduct and dissemination of the studies they founded. "One of the Bay-Dole legacies has been to expose medical science to the corrupt influence of...[corporations]. (p. 74,75) Both DSM and Bay-Dole [have] create the perfect storm for more children to take more drugs more often" (p.75). (Bakan also points out that SSRIs (except Prozac) are forbidden in Britain.)

19. Parent Involvement and Law Suits

There have been several law suits in which parents fought either the prescription of psychotropic drugs for their children or where parent groups sued the makers of these drugs.

The "Tribune Review" (no date available) reported the case <u>Senatore v. Senatore</u>". The article says:

> "a father sued his child's mother after she took her son to a therapist who prescribed an antidepressant to curb his aggressive behavior. The father's objection was that the medication was not proven to be safe for kids. In addition, he argued that the divorced parents shared legal custody, and that the mother had no right to make this decision alone. Ruling for the father, a family court judge decided that the mother's unilateral decision to place the son on the medication deprived the father of his right to equal participation in major decision [sic] impacting his son's life. The court directed that the prescription medicine be discontinued until the parties agreed on a course of behavior."

The writer remarks, that "In this month's "Pennsylvania Lawyer", attorney Dr. Nora Porter notes

> that an increasing number of plaintiffs may join class action lawsuits filed last year alleging damage to children by the drug <u>Ritalin</u>. These lawsuits charge defendants <u>Novartis,</u> the drug manufacturer, <u>Children and Adults with Attention Deficit Disorder</u> and the <u>American Psychiatric Association</u> with conspiracy to overpromote the diagnosis of Attention Deficit Hyperactivity Disorder. The lawsuits charge that the defendants willfully failed to provide adequate information to consumers, doctors and schools concerning the hazards of the drug. The result, said Porter, is <u>that school authorities, law enforcement personnel, lawyers and courts have ended up encouraging or forcing Ritalin on kids who are acting up...</u>"

Porter noted that Ritalin is categorized by the Drug Enforcement Administration as a Schedule II drug…Ritalin's listed side effects include addiction, loss of appetite, difficulty sleeping, depression, confusion, robotic or obsessive-compulsive behavior, aggression and hostility, Tourette's syndrome, mania, hallucinations and more. "

The article lists two websites to learn about the litigation:

- www.edforce.house.gove/hearings/106th/01/ritalin92900
- www.ritalin-fraud.com

Another case is described by <u>Alexandra Marks,</u> staff writer for the Christian Science Monitor (Oct.6, 2000). In this case, a father, Michael <u>Caroll,</u> had taken his son off Ritalin. For this, he had been reported by the local school district. (The article points out that the use of the drug has increased 700 percent in the last decade.) The father claimed that the drug had "turned the once-rambunctious boy into a withdrawn insomniac with no appetite. And his reading level, which was the original cause of Carrol's concern, had not improved." The article states that the case is not unique and

> that educators, psychologists and a "medical community" appear to be convinced that the drug helps children. There have been congressional hearings, proposals for a national policy and several class action lawsuits.

The writer quotes Peter Breggin:

> "The drugging of children has gotten so out of hand…This is a national catastrophe. I'm seeing children who are normal who are on five psychiatric drugs."

 Marks continues: After child welfare officials told Caroll to put his son back on Ritalin or risk losing custody, Kyle resumed taking the drug. But this summer, a judge ruled that if Caroll could find another doctor to say that Ritalin was unnecessary, Kyle [his son] could stop taking it. Caroll succeeded. Since August, Kyle has not used Ritalin." The writer quotes the author of "Running on Ritalin", <u>Lawrence Diller,</u> who says that there is a "growing cultural acceptance "of a misperception, namely that physiological factors are responsible for "children's misbehavior and underperformance." He feels that there are other strategies to handle these problems, but that that would take more time, effort and money. The writer continues:

> "…class-action lawsuits in California and New Jersey brought last month, accuse the maker of Ritalin and APA of worse than expedience. They claim the two conspired to create a market for the drug by concocting the ADHD diagnosis and putting out pamphlets in schools that touted the drug's effectiveness without advising that is has "no long-term effect "in improving academic performance or in helping kids overcome hyperactivity."

 The writer points out the <u>Frasers</u> of Rockville, Md. Their son Andrew has a high I.Q. A second grade teacher recommended treating him for ADHD. He was put on Ritalin, had problems sleeping and ended up being on four drugs. ("Side effects of one drug were addressed by prescribing additional drugs.")

The Frasers took their son off the drugs. He is doing well and they wish they had never put him on the drugs, but instead had looked at their family dynamics and made some important changes in this regard.

Another class action suit against a pharmaceutical company was the <u>Wesbecker</u> trial that I mentioned in chapter 2 and 20.

Yet another class- action suit was brought by the families of five students who were killed in the Columbine High School shooting. The antidepressant <u>Luvox</u> was found in the dead shooter's body. The law-suit claimed that the company that makes Luvox, Solvay, failed to warn Harris' doctors about the side effects. "Such drugs caused Eric Harris to become manic and psychotic", the law-suit stated. (s. chapter 2.)

20. The science behind antipsychotics

In the following, I will try to explain the scientific background for these drugs by using <u>Dr. Joseph Glenmullen's</u> book <u>"Prozac backlash."</u> (2000) (Glenmullen is a clinical instructor in psychiatry at Harvard Medical school.) He cites Sherwin Nuland, professor of surgery and historian of medicine at Yale (in the New York Review of books) who says that the public is being

> "subjected to the arguments of seemingly authoritative physicians and scientists...it remains anything but certain that clinical depression is caused by a decrease in serotonin deficiencies and biochemical imbalance" (p.15)..."Half a million children are prescribed the drugs. This in spite of the fact that repeated studies have shown that antidepressant drugs are no more effective in children than placebos." (p.15)

He continues and explains brain chemistry:

> Brain chemicals are called neurotransmitters. There are more than 100 known. Serotonin, adrenalin and dopamine are referred to as the "feel good" neurotransmitters. Cocaine and amphetamines boost all three neurotransmitters. [The] Prozac group was hailed as a breakthrough because it was "selective" for serotonin. This selectivity gives the impression that serotonin is localized in the depression center in the brain. If a depressed person's serotonin is low, the impression is given that the drugs top it up in a safe targeted manner. This impression does not match reality." (p.16) "There is no depression center in the brain. Rather the drugs have global effects owing to Serotonin's vast influence." (p.17) "In humans only 5 % of serotonin is found in the brain. The other 95 % is distributed throughout the rest of the body (in the gastro-intestinal tract, the cardiovascular system, blood clotting, influence on the genitals. (This explains the side effects of painful long erection in young boys. (s. FDA warning forRitalin) "It plays a significant role in controlling a host of hormones that regulate a panoply of physiologic processes." (p.16)

Glenmullen explains:

> Serotonin is a chemical by which the brain cells communicate with each other. Serotonin nerves originate in the brain stem. It is the largest brain system known.

 He cites Efrain Azmitia, professor of biology and psychiatry at New York University and one of the world's leading authors on Serotonin :

> "Serotonin has been implicated in sleep, aggression, sexual activity, appetite, learning and memory, to name just a few behaviors altered by Serotonin drugs or damage to the 5-HT (serotonin nerve) fibers." (p.16)

<u>Wikipedia</u> explains how the SSRIs work:

> " In the brain, messages are passed from a nerve cell to another via a chemical synapse, a small gap between the cells. The ...cell that sends the information releases neurotransmitters including serotonin into the gap. The neurotransmitters are then recognized by receptors on the surface of the recipient...cell, which..., in turn, relays the signal ...90% are released from the receptors and taken up again by ...transporters into the sending... cell, a process called *reuptake.*

> SSRIs inhibit the reuptake of serotonin. As a result, serotonin stays in the...gap longer and may repeatedly stimulate the receptors of the recipient cell." (on7.3.24)

Glenmullen states that this leads to artificially elevated serotonin levels. (p.20.) (Remember: Depression and other mental disorders are supposedly caused by low serotonin levels.)

Boosting Serotonin can trigger compensatory changes in the other neurotransmitters (e.g. a drop in dopamine) which doctors and scientist are just beginning to understand. "The connections between the serotonin and dopamine systems in the brain are thought to be responsible for drugs' severe effects." (p.20). Glenmullen calls this the "Prozac backlash" but states that this observation applies to other drugs, also. He remarks that the FDA approval process (that is so important to many people) only assures short term safety, "typically only for 6 -8 weeks whereas <u>the most serious long-term side effects … take years, sometimes decades to emerge."</u> (p. 20)

Glenmullen states that Ely- Lilly has denied that suicides and violence are side effects and he cites the case of Joseph Wesbecker. (s. chapter 2) He writes that because the long-term effects are not studied:

> <u>"Under these circumstances, prescribing an entirely new class of agents to millions of people is nothing short of an ongoing human experiment"</u>

and he quotes Professor of Psychiatry and Neuroscience, Ross Baldessari:

> <u>"Man is becoming the primary guinea pig."</u> (p.20/21)

He continues: "Regrettably, in the current climate, many people are put on the drugs indefinitely…patients are often not told about withdrawal which can be severe…In the early 1990, when Prozac's dangerous effects surfaced in the media, the FDA asked a special committee to look into the matter of suicidality and violence and turned to a panel of "independent (meaning outside of the FDA), blue ribbon experts. "In this case there were nine doctors, <u>five of whose financial ties to pharmaceutical companies</u> – including the manufacturers of serotonin boosters required waivers of its own standards regarding conflicts of interest."(p.156,157)

There were hearings about this on September 20, 1991. Fifty members of the public were allowed to address the committee and speak for five minutes. "Some were patients who told how they had become suicidal and violent on Prozac. Others were family members of people who had committed suicide… A number of psychiatrists and drug proponents [warned] the committee, that any changes in the prescribing guidelines would undermine the public's interest in psychiatric drugs." (p. 157)

The FDA staff explained that

> there is no systematic program for monitoring side effects of drugs once they are on the market.

"Suicide and violence… may need further investigation… and does not itself constitute evidence of causality."(p.158) The committee members voted unanimously that antidepressants do not cause suicide and violence. One third of the panel members voted for a warning on the labels. They were outvoted by two thirds who were against it. Glenmullen writes:

> "By 1991 Prozac was already the number- one bestselling antidepressant, with sales near one billion a year…So the pharmaceutical industry and the drug advocates decided to defend Prozac at all costs, despite the risk to individual and public safety. "(p.161)

"More than 150 Prozac lawsuits had already been filed by December 1994 (p. 173). Glenmullen cites Harvard Medical School psychiatrist Martin Teicher who reported that Prozac could induce "intense, violent suicidal preoccupation" (p.135) and "We know that some of these drugs can produce a worsening or exacerbation in anxiety, at least initially and sometimes they can induce panic attacks. (In Germany, the prescription guidelines for Prozak warn of suicidality.)

Glenmullen continues:

> "In the last decade, around the country, communities have been shocked by brutal, senseless murders and murder- suicides. How many of these sensational tragedies might have been due to serotonin boosters. Should doctors and families, left guilt ridden over events of suicide or violence committed by a patient or family member, be considering the possibility that a serotonin booster may be responsible? How often might Prozac, Zoloft, Paxil or Luvox have been the missing clue, the secret that would help explain suicides or murder – suicides that have been devastating to families, caregivers and communities?"(p. 186) Glenmullen also points out

<u>"The United States is the only country in the world where potent, synthetic drugs targeting the brain are routinely prescribed for children"</u>. (p.130)

In this regard <u>Dr. Christiane Northrupp</u>, in her book "The Wisdom of Menopause" (2006) says the following:

"There are apt to be side effects from the long-term of any drug that alters brain chemistry and many of the popular psychotic drugs on the market today are too new for anybody to say with authority that they are safe in the long run."(p. 327, 328)

<u>Candace Pert</u>, the scientist who discovered the receptor side for many important chemicals in the brain associated with mood, commented in her book "Molecules of Emotions"(1997):

" I am alarmed at the monster that Johns Hopkins neuroscientist Solomon Snyder and I created when we discovered the simple binding assay for drug reception 25 years ago. Prozac and other antidepressant serotonin –receptor-active compounds may also cause cardiovascular problems in some susceptible people after long-term use, which has become common practice despite the lack of safety studies. The public is being misinformed about the precision of the SSRIs."

Pert explains how the medications work:

A receptor, a single molecule, is floating on the cell membrane made up of proteins (amino acids). It has roots reaching in to the interior of a cell. A typical nerve cell (neuron) may have millions of receptors on its surface. Their chemical structure can now be identified. Receptors are sensing molecules scanners. They hover in the membrane waiting to pick up messages carried by other vibrating little creatures (amino acids) that cruise through the fluid surrounding the cell. We think of them as keyholes, which is not correct because they constantly move and vibrate. All the receptors are proteins. They wait in the membrane for the right chemical keys to swim up to them and to mount them by fitting into their keyhole (ligand), i.e. exactly right shape. (binding) The ligand is the chemical key that binds to the receptor, enters it like a key in a keyhole, creates a disturbance to tickle the molecule into rearranging itself changing its shape until...information enters its cell. (p.23 ff.) The receptor, after it received a message transmits it into the cell interior where the message can change the state of the cell dramatically. Any number of activities can be started: manufacturing of proteins, cell divisions, opening and closing ion channels, adding or subtracting chemical groups like phosphates. They can translate into changes in behavior, physical activity, mood. (p.24)

Pert points out that the process of binding is very selective. The receptor ignores all but the specific ligand. For instance, the opiate receptor can only receive ligands of the opiate group.

Ligands consists of 3 chemical types

1. Neurotransmitters, like dopamine, histamine, Gaba and serotonin
2. Steroids
3. Peptides (make up 95% of ligands and regulate practically all life processes and are amino acids like the receptors.)

Pert compares the cell to an engine, receptors to buttons on a control panel and ligands to a finger that pushes the button to get things started.

She informs us that in the early 20th century scientists found new chemical substances, the neurotransmitters in the brain and that the first receptor was isolated in a lab in 1972. Scientists concluded that if a drug worked that there had to be a receptor for this drug. To find out which were neurotransmitters: measure the reuptake mechanism = <u>the excess juices left over after binding would be sucked back into the neuron and destroyed.</u> Now it would be possible to measure the receptor. Two nearly identical drugs could bind to the same receptor:

1. The agonist could enter the receptor and create changes in the cell.
2. The antagonist could block the same receptor and no observable changes in the cell would occur.
3. Pert wanted to use Naloxone as an antagonist. She assumed that it could bump heroin from its receptor, displacing it and then occupy the receptor site itself. She discovered the opiate receptor on Oct. 25, 2072.

It was found that endorphin was the body's own natural morphine that uses the opiate receptor. It is located in the brain and its ligand fits into the opiate receptor and creates the same effects like opiates.

So an endogenous substance was discovered that fit into the body's opiate receptor. (p.70). It was a peptide produced in the brain and had its receptor in the brain. Pain relief was mediated in the brain. Every peptide was a candidate for a brain receptor search to investigate how they interacted with the brain to cause many bodily functions. In 1973 it was discovered that the opiate receptors were most dense in the limbic system of the brain (seat of emotional circuitry.) The race to find the chemical structures of the brain's natural opiates was on.

Later in her book Pert describes to a counsellor the chemical action of the psychotropic drugs: "The brain cells communicate with each other across the synapse. Chemicals are squirted out by one and bind to the receptor of another. "If there is too much a reuptake mechanism comes into play, that is, the cell reabsorbs the excess." The classical understanding of depression is that there is a shortage of...serotonin secreted by the brain cells. To remedy this, the antidepressant drug is used to block the reuptake mechanism, allowing the excess serotonin to flood the receptors and thereby correct the imbalance." (p.266, 267) What doesn't get measured is what else is going on in other parts of the brain and body where these drugs get administered. "Your intestines, for instance, are loaded with serotonin receptors just as cells in the immune system which could influence the growth of cancer cells."

" Often people on antidepressants have gastrointestinal disorders." So medication like Haldol, Thorazine, Risperdal, Clorazil block receptors for dopamine. The author states :" When dopamine receptors in the pituitary glands of women are blocked, women stop menstruating, are in a constant state of PMS complete with water retention and weight gain. Often these women are given antidepressants."

Peter Breggin explains the chemistry behind the SSRIs more closely in his book "Talking back to Prozac" (1998). He writes:

"Prozac, Zoloft and Paxil are described as "selective" uptake blockers. That is they are supposed to impact on seratonergic nerves with little or no spread of effect to other transmitter systems or brain functions." (p.24) He states that this is not so. "The SSRIs end up heavily impacting other neurotransmitter systems. One of Prozac's most menacing side effects is probably due to its effect on dopamine.("Serotonergic nerves spread like a branching tree throughout the brain and spinal cord. The axoms of serotonergic cell bodies affect other nerves that control bodily functions. Serotonin is, in fact, the most widespread neurotransmitter system in the brain. (p.25.) He writes:

"No one prescribing or receiving the drug can fully grasp Prozac's overall impact on the brain and whole body, because it's beyond our current scientific understanding."(p. 26)

He continues:

"The brain is made up several hundred billion neurons and trillions of synapses… the biochemical activities that run the brain remain almost wholly shrouded in mystery. We have no idea… how the brain makes a thought or an emotion. It seems foolhardy to imagine that blocking one of the brain's biochemical functions would somehow improve the brain and the mind." (p.39) He claims that it is "a dangerous assumption that it is safe and effective to tamper with the most complex organ in the universe" (p.40) He concludes:

"All the FDA drug studies are constructed, supervised and paid for by the drug companies themselves, using doctors and research teams of their own choosing-often people who have long-established relationships with the company. "(p.41)

21. Suppression of negative results

You can find the following information on Wikipedia (accessed on 7.3.2024) under
Antidepressants : "A study examining publication of results from FDA- evaluated
antidepressants concluded that those with favorable results were much more
likely to be published than those with negative results. Furthermore, an
investigation of 185 meta analysis on antidepressants found that 79% of them
had authors affiliated in some way to pharmaceutical companies and that they
were reluctant to report caveats for antidepressants." (footnotes under nos. 194,
195)

      Mildred K. Cho of the Center for Bioethics at the University of Pennsylvania
and Lisa A. Bero of the University of California reported their findings –

> that symposia (papers published in medical journals) sponsored up to
> 70 % by drug companies tended to use misleading titles and lacked
> reviews by independent experts. They also omitted often an
> explanation of how the research was conducted and therefore
> depriving the public of a critical evaluation. (published in the Annals
> of Internal Medicine)

(The Washington Post, published by the Tribune Review, March 17, 1996)

      Not always is there a suppression of negative results, but these are often
whitewashed. Eli Lilly, e.g. warned that their ADHD drug Strattera could cause
suicidal thoughts on patients. The FDA is planning (or did) to add a warning label
to this drug. Dr. John R.R. Hayes, vice president of Lilly Research Laboratories
remarked "This kInd of label information in no way precludes prescribing
(Strattera)". The article I am quoting is stating that Strattera was Lilly's sixth bestselling drug last year (2005) with $667 million in sales. "The warning comes after
Lilly responded to an FDA request to reanalyze its data on 1,357 children and
adolescents who took Strattera in placebo-controlled clinical trials...Five children,
or 0.4 percent reported suicidal thoughts while taking the drug, including one
child who attempted suicide....In a control group...none had suicidal thoughts."
Dr. Hayes concluded "Strattera continues to be a safe and effective treatment
option." (Jeff Swiatek in "The Indianapolis Star" quoted in the "Tribune Review",
Sept.30, 2005)

Another article warns:

> "Reports of psychosis or mania in children were associated with all of the increasingly popular drugs used to treat attention-deficit-hyperactivity disorder, federal health officials say in documents released as an advisory panel prepares to consider stronger warning labels...The reviews show that the adverse events, particularly hallucinations (involving insects, snakes and worms), can occur in some patients at normal doses of any ADHD drug. The reviews included about 90 studies of the drugs as well as reports from doctors, parents and others. The ADHD drugs include Ritalin, Adderall ...and Strattera. "The FDA also considered further warning about possible problems like heart attack, stroke and hypertension.

(Andrew Bridges from the Associated Press, quoted in the Tribune Review, March 22, 2006)

Wayne Condro writes for the Canadian Medical Association (CMAJ , March 02, 2004:

> " An internal document advised staff at ...GlaxoSmithKline (GSK) to withhold clinical trial findings in 1998 that indicated the antidepressant paroxetine (Paxil) ...had no beneficial effect in treating adolescents.."

The article claims that the US and Canada has since banned the drug for pediatric use because of increased risk of suicide. Canada issued a public warning that the pediatric use drugs of Paroxetine, Wellbutrin, Celexa, Luvox, Remeron, Zoloft and Effexor "should proceed only after consultation with the treating physician." An internal document obtained by CMAJ "provides guidance on how to manage the results of 2 clinical trials conducted into the efficacy of paroxetine." The clinical trials were "insufficiently robust" to achieve approval of Seroxat (name used in the UK) for use in pediatric depression. The author points out that the sale of Seroxat amounted to almost $4.97 billion worldwide in 2003. Studies carried out in the US and elsewhere showed that a placebo "was actually more effective than the antidepressant." He writes:

> "Britain's Medicines and Healthcare Products Regulatory Authority (MHRA) advised doctors in June 2003 that paroxetine should not be prescribed to patients under the age of 18 because evidence from various clinical trials showed that episodes of suicidal behavior were

between 1.5 and 3.2 times higher in children taking the drug than in those receiving placebo. Several nations, including the US, France and Ireland quickly followed suit." He claims the FDA is now reviewing pediatric trials of 8 antidepressants. He says that it has been estimated that as many as 11 million and 3 million Canadian children are taking antidepressants.

The Lancet, the highly regarded English medical journal, wrote in an editorial (Volume 363, Number 9418):

"It is hard to imagine the anguish experienced by the parents, relatives and friends of a child who has taken his or her own life. That such an event could be precipitated by a supposedly beneficial drug is a catastrophe. The idea of this drug's use being based on the selective reporting of favourable research should be unimaginable. In this week's issue of the Lancet (p. 1341), however, a meta-analysis by Craig Whittington and colleagues suggests that this is what has been happening for research into the use of antidepressants in childhood. Their results illustrates an abuse of the trust patients place in their physicians....The story of research into selective serotonin reuptake inhibitor (SSRI) use in childhood depression is one of confusion, manipulation and institutional failure. Although published evidence was inconsistent at best, use of SSRIs to treat childhood depression has been encouraged by pharmaceutical companies and clinicians worldwide. "

The article mentions the internal memorandum by GlaxoSmithKline that I mentioned above concerning paroxetine, that states "it would be unacceptable to include a statement that efficacy has not been demonstrated, as this would undermine the profile of paroxetine."

The authors criticize the FDA for not acting appropriately on information provided to them that these drugs were ineffective and harmful to children. The article asks for changes for the healthcare infrastructure. The authors write:

"people around the world ...will not ...tolerate the notion that in biomedical research this could be at the expense of their children's lives."

In an article by the researcher E. <u>Jane Garland</u> in the CMAJ (Canadian Medical Association in 2004) the author criticizes the use of paroxetine similar to the criticism above, but also adds the drug <u>venlafaxine</u> to the list of dangerous drugs because of its ineffectiveness and doubling the rate of suicidality and hostility. Compared to a placebo. (She uses important references in her article). She states:

> " A general advisory was…issued regarding the increased risks of suicide in pediatric use of *all* SSRIs. These developments not only raise new concerns about the presumed effectiveness and safety of SSRIs for young people, but also pose disturbing questions about publication bias and the questionable interpretation of research data on the treatment of childhood depression."

The author states that

> <u>"observations in clinical trials and case reports indicate that up to 25% of children placed on SSRIs for any disorder will experience other psychiatric adverse effects including agitation, irritability and behavioral disinhibition</u>. In the adolescent paroxetine trial, 10.5% of patients discontinued paroxetine because of "serious "psychiatric adverse effects… Such responses led 7.5% of the outpatient participants prescribed paroxetine who initially were only mildly depressed to be admitted to hospital, while none of the placebo group required hospital admission,…the fact, that researchers have minimized these adverse events underscores concerns about the complex <u>conflicts of interest</u> that may affect the conduct, analysis and reporting of clinical trials."

The author mentioned a sertraline trial that did not include a side effect checklist, "yet the medication was listed as well tolerated." She states that many physicians find it difficult "to accept that SSRIs may be ineffective." She continues that the physician treating a child or adolescent with onset of depression should begin with "nonpharmacological therapies " but might use an SSRI that has been approved for children. She warns, however:

> "Physicians need to be alert to the fact that the psychiatric adverse effects of SSRIs overlap with manifestations of depression itself; without this realization, physicians may make the mistake of increasing rather than decreasing the SSRI dose of children

experiencing these adverse effects, or of unnecessarily prescribing adjunctive mood stabilizers and atypical neuroleptics."

She warns of the dangers of withdrawal from the SSRIs. She also points out that young patients and their parents don't realize that SSRIs do not cure depression, but "might improve some depressive symptoms." She closes by stating:

> "Publication of all clinical trials results and systematic ascertainment of adverse effects must become research standards. Furthermore, data must be subject to analysis by independent experts who are alert to conflicts of interest that may distort the interpretation of data. Practice guidelines need to be rewritten to reflect a critical analysis of the full body of evidence, both published and unpublished."

In his book "Your drug might be the problem" (1999), Peter Breggin writes that the FDA is largely dependent on the information the drug companies provide. He states:

> "Management of the company headquarters makes the final decision about how to handle the data submitted to it by its paid researchers. If management decides that there is no possible connection between the company's drug and the patient's negative reaction, the data may never find its way to the FDA". (p. (101)

He continues:

> "Through the Freedom of Information Act (FOIA) any citizen can obtain a summary of pre-marketing drug testing results for a specific medication... But the basic underlying data...are the secret property of the drug company. Only a product liability suit against Pfizer would open access to the company's own research records. Some drug companies actually settle product liability suits against them. Physicians and even key health policy planners do not have access to all the necessary data required to make an independent evaluation of a drug's safety. They must instead rely on very general information provided by the FDA, which in turn relies largely on the drug companies." (p. 102)

He writes:

"FDA records contain thousands of reports of severe and life-threatening reactions to almost every psychiatric drug in current use. With respect to each of these drugs, the agency has attempted to determine, if, on balance, it is sufficiently useful to outweigh its potential dangers. But this evaluation does not necessarily mean that the drug is safe. Indeed, determination of whether the drug's potential benefits outweigh its potential risks is, of necessity, highly subjective. Hence, FDA approval should not be interpreted as indicating that a given drug is without serious and potentially fatal adverse reactions. On the contrary, all psychiatric drugs approved by the FDA can pose enormous risks even in routine use." (p.102)

22. Children in foster care, veterans, the homeless, prisoners and the elderly

According to the Government's Center for Disease Control and Prevention (https://www.cdc.gov, in 2019, 13.6 % of U.S. children between the ages of 5 and 17 years had received mental health treatment in the past 12 months...8.4% had taken prescription drug psychotropics. According to "Psychology today" (posted on August 17, 2021) 1.2% of preschoolers were taking these drugs and according to the "Center for Health Statistics" 16.5 adults were taking psychotropics in 2020. The National Institute of Health (NIH).gov. (no year listed) stated that 17 % of men and 48 % of women in prison were on psychotropic drugs. The homeless are often prescribed these drugs ("street medicine"-which provides medical care for the "unsheltered"), but it is difficult to find out how many. According to the PCORI (Patient- Centered Outcomes Research Institute (https://www.pcori.org) an independent non-profit research organization created to help patients and those who care for them, partially funded by the government and insurance companies), one out of four children in foster care were given these drugs, often a combination of two, three or four drugs. The authors of this report state that

> "monitoring of children administered psychotropic medication is infrequent and often fails to follow professional guidelines...Often these drugs are prescribed without clarity as to who is authorized to consent and without procedure that protects the foster youth."

Linda Britton is a lawyer and directs the ABA commission on Youth at Risk. writes in the "American Bar Association:" (April 01, 2016) under the title "Limiting psochotropic medication and improving mental health treatment for children in custody." (her here expressed views have not (regrettably) been approved by the American Bar Association). She reports about the increase of prescribed psychotropic medication "those substances that act upon the brain to chemically alter mood, cognition and behavior" in the general population, but a higher increase in children and youth who are poor. She writes that the highest use is in children and youth in foster care, in residential group homes, in treatment centers and in juvenile detention centers. She points out that:

> "Lawyers who represent children in the child welfare and/or juvenile
> justice system should know that large numbers of children ...are
> prescribed these medications   without... the procedures parents
> would insist upon...and with minimal oversight by those charged ...to
> act in the best interest of the child" because of the health risks
> involved.

She continues:

> "The psychotropic medications ...are often administered for "off-
> label" use, in amounts that often exceeds recommended dosages,
> and often in combination with other psychotropic medications as a
> first resort instead of a last one".

She lists the short – term side effects of increased heart-rate and blood pressure,
weight gain, sleepiness, sedation, tremor, anxiety, dizziness , confusion and
changes in behavior and seizure. "Long –term effects are completely unknown".
She writes:

> "Children and youths repeatedly complain that psychotropic
> medications make them "feel like zombies", unable to function in
> school and uninterested in outside activities.

The author lists several children with a foster care background who were on
different psychotropic medications, up, in some cases to 12, sometimes on four or
five at the same time. One young girl who had been physically and mentally
abused was prescribed powerful psychotropic medication to numb her pain. "She
was so medicated... that she literally lost her ability to speak."
The author also sees a danger in the fact, that psychotropic drugs "mask
children's symptoms and offer a quick fix." She writes:

> "In many cases these drugs are prescribed without a full medical
> history, a full evaluation and diagnosis...In other words, medical
> protocols and procedures that protect the rights of patients are
> absent."

Briton urges attorneys and judges involved in the child welfare and juvenile
justice system to use national practice guidelines and policy resolutions. She
points out that

"Several national organizations, including most recently the American Bar Association have issued [those] to improve oversight and procedures in cases where children are prescribed psychotropic medication. These are useful resources for child advocates and can add weight to arguments raising concerns about psychotropic medication in "children.""

She also names the American Academy of Child and Adolescent Psychiatrists who have written guidelines for this purpose. These guidelines include the following:

- No psychotropic drug should be prescribed without the informed consent by the child, the parent[s], guardian or licensed caretaker. States should identify each involved party "that is empowered to consent for treatment" for children under the age of fourteen. At age fourteen, the child should decide for himself.

- No psychotropic medication should be prescribed without appropriate administration, oversight and regulation. Short and long monitoring plans are essential to assess developments or increases in suicidal ideation, initial side effect and potential changes over time.

- No dosages should be exceeded, no off-label use should be applied and no combination with other drugs should be permitted without "secondary review".

Alternative therapies should be used before or at the same time that these drugs are administered.

The author also points out that "The National Council of Juvenile and Family Court Judges" passed a resolution in July 2013

urging courts to improve supervision and oversight of medical and mental health issues including the use of psychotropic medication, of children and youth under their jurisdiction."

She writes that the American Bar Association approved a resolution in February 2016 that asked the child welfare and juvenile justice agencies, among other things, to use means to reduce the "need to prescribe psychotropic drugs." And to avoid the use these drugs "solely to control behavior", that lawyers involved "should become fully educated" about the rights of these children and juveniles and that states will be able to report to the appropriate federal agencies about these issues, "so that progress can be demonstrated."

Briton also feels that states and administrative agencies involved must protect children in state custody from over-medication. Oversight protocols should be implemented to manage and regulate the use of psychotropics. The author bemoans the fact, that lawyers and judges involved often just accept the prescription for the children as medically necessary (and best being left to the "experts".) She urges these legal entities to ask the following questions "at a minimum":

- Why is this prescribed?'
- Why is this amount necessary?
- Where can I learn more about this medication and its side effects?
- What are the possible long term consequences of use of this medication?
- Who has informed consent on this decision and has he/she given consent?
- What other treatments and therapies exist for this diagnosis?
- How will this medication be monitored?

(See, http://www.americanbar.org/groups/youth at risk.html)

"Psychology Today,"posted August 17, 2021:

> "Very little is known about the effects of these drugs taken alone or in combination on the developing brain. Most of the prescribing is "off label", meaning essentially unlicensed and with unproven efficacy and safety."

In regard to suicides among <u>veterans,</u> the "U.S. Pharmacist", a publication for pharmacists, writes on Nov. 17, 2016 in its abstract:

> "In 2014, the office of Suicide Prevention of the US Department of Veterans' Affairs reported that veterans have a 21% higher risk for

suicides (in NEWS provided by EIN Presswire (Press release distribution service (https://www.einpresswire.com))

On Nov. 10, 2022, it is stated:

> Of the 9 million U.S. veterans enrolled in VA health services in 1919, 4.2 million were prescribed psychiatric drugs. When compared to civilian adults…possessing knowledge of medications associated with an increased risk of suicide…can equip pharmacists with the tools needed to help suicides in this population."

Under Medications with increased risk of Suicidality they write that

> the FDA has identified over 125 drugs for potential increased risk of suicidal ideation and behavior and that it enforces BBWs (Black box warnings) for these medications. Patients on antidepressants should be monitored. Pharmacists should help identify at risk-patients and should engage in discussions regarding suicide because of their role in dispensing mental health medication. Pharmacies should watch out for changes in medication. They should watch with drugs with BBWs (suicidality) have been prescribed. They also should warn of the dangers of abrupt discontinuation of these drugs.

(Abuse of psychiatric drugs in the elderly, especially in nursing homes, is widespread and requires urgent examination and changes that, however, go beyond the limits of this book.)

23. The role of government

The government requests parity, i.e. equality of treatment for physical and mental ailments as written in the <u>2008 Mental Health and Addiction Parity Act for Large Health Group Plans.</u> That means that some insurers pay if a patient is admitted to a psychiatric unit. The coverage varies with smaller health insurance companies. With them it is often harder to prove when mental health treatment is needed. They often require that the cheapest method is used first. So, it's a good idea to check with your insurer what is covered under your policy.

<u>Medicare</u> looks, for instance, for indications of mental disorders like sad, empty, hopeless feelings, lack of energy, troubles sleeping, etc. for a diagnosis for depression.

Medicare pays for in- and outpatient services.

Part B covers visits with psychiatrists, physician's assistants, nurse practitioners etc. There is a Medicare deductible. It covers a yearly depression screening, psychotherapy, family counselling, prescription, partial hospitalization and medication. The Medicare drug plans have to cover antidepressants, anticonvulsants and antipsychotic medication. (if you have a limited income and resources, you may qualify for "Extra Help")

In most states, individuals who have a mental illness are eligible for <u>SSI (Supplemental Security Insurance).</u>

     <u>Medicaid</u> is the single largest payer for mental health services. (According to a White House publication on May 31, 2022 the government spends \$280 billion on mental health yearly)

The government states that 11 % of youth have been diagnosed with a mental illness.

Medicaid.gov states:

> "Children exposed to trauma have the same symptoms like children in treatment. Family violence and neglect exhibit symptoms that are consistent with individuals diagnosed with post traumatic stress disorder, attention deficit hyper activity disorder, depression and conduct disorder/oppositional defiant disorder."

The article claims:

"The presence of major depression, bipolar disorder and alcohol and
drug abuse are frequent risk factors for suicidal behavior."
<u>(no mention is made of the side effects of psychotropic medication)</u>

In the introduction to the handbook "Using Medicaid to Support Working Age Adults with Serious Mental Illnesses in the Community ", current as of January 2005, published by the government, it is stated "There are now effective medications' evidence based…"(There is no indication of the dangers when using these medications!) The handbook also points out the high cost of treatment, but does not mention the huge financial gains for the pharmaceutical industry that is, of course, borne by the taxpayer.)

Let's take a look at <u>SSI payments</u>. The General Accounting Office (GAO), a government entity (no date avail.) stated: "At the end of 2022 the average SSI payment that Social Security paid for children was $732."

On AI overview you can read "according to the National survey of SSI children and families, about 36 percent of children receiving SSI have a mental disability. The 2022 SSI Annual Statistical Report also states that six out of 10 recipients under age 65 have a mental disease."

The Washington Post wrote (on February 4, 1994) an article with the title: "Cost soar for children's disability program." The author writes: "Under a broad new federal standard prompted by a 1990 Supreme Court ruling, behavior that isn't 'age appropriate' is considered to be a disability."

There is a real danger of parents enrolling their children into this program in order to receive SSI payments. (s. Bruce Levine's description of the case of Rebeccah Riley.)

24. Financial background and the corporate take-over of our health system

There are several very important phenomena that do not only influence, but dominate our health system, including psychotropic drugs.

In 1984 <u>Stanley Wohl,</u> M.D. wrote a seminal book about our health-system and the changes that are occurring in this system with the title <u>"The Medical Industrial Complex."</u>(1984). He describes the emergence "of a major new American industry, corporate medicine" (p.1) He is careful to point out that some effects of corporate power are positive (like cost containment and uniform standards as the for profit systems claim.) (p.2) He, however, describes his dismay when he finds out that the heads of hospitals now can be businessmen and public relations executive. (p.5) He feels that "unregulated business-medicine marriage "spelled "disaster for the moral and ethical foundation for…" medicine. (p.6)

In the book, Wohl describes the beginning of the corporization of medicine by naming a doctor, Thomas Frist, who, for the first time, sold shares in a hospital to be able to raise capital. The author calls the year 1965 a watershed in his story when the U.S. Congress passed the Medicare and Medicaid entitlement programs for the elderly and the poor, with Medicaid paying for the poor and disabled of any age. Health care costs increased rapidly. Corporations and doctors began to realize that the reimbursement were very generous. ("Medicare mills" p.8) Soon Dr. Frist founded the Hospital Corporation of America. The hospital controlled eleven hospitals, fifteen years later almost four hundred. (p.9) Other medical entrepreneurs followed. As Wohl states "The formula in all cases were very nearly the same: study the Medicare legislation; form a corporation; go public to raise capital; acquire more and more health care facilities; and make a healthy profit for all concerned." (p. 9, 10)

Wohl describes another entrepreneur who ran into financial troubles but was able to convince a large Southern investment firm, Stephen's Inc., to buy a large block of that company's stock. Later, companies like Dow Chemical, Monsanto and Standard Oil "were either buying shares in the newly formed health provider firms or themselves setting up health provider divisions." (p.11)

"Since many of these conglomerates were previously medical suppliers" the distinction between medical suppliers and medical providers did not exist any longer. Soon corporate America acquired medical groups, hospitals, nursing homes, Urgent Care –type facilities and free-standing surgery centers. Wohl states that "at the present" (1984) there were about five hundred listed corporations who compete for healthcare investments. (p.15) (According to the US Census Bureau from Oct. 14, 2020 there were 907,426 corporations involved in healthcare and social assistance.) Their profit amounts to 22.4 billion according to Beck's Hospital Review, March 7, 2024.

Wohl states that in the last twenty years (again, the book was published in 1984) there were two very important trends in healthcare: a huge increase in cost and a great increase in corporations who provide health care. (The profit for the corporations is one third!) (p.17) "The growing corporate ownership of hospital chains and physician groups is at the heart of the…Medical Industrial Complex…MIC." (p.18) As of 1983, corporations owned 11% of the nation's 5,900 community hospitals and 66% of nursing homes. (p.19) Wohl points out how expenditure has changed. In the past, the majority of dollars were spent on doctors or surgeons but now it is spent on ancillary costs: hospital beds, drugs, lab tests, expensive medical equipment etc. "Of $1.00 spent on health, only $0.02 now ends up with the physician. (p.19) (The NIH (National Institute of Health) claims, that it is 10%. (Jan./Feb. 2013) And of the $317 billion spent on healthcare in 1982, fully $118 billion turned up as corporate revenues… It's a multibillion business the employs ten million Americans." … (p. 19, 20)

Wohl lists 6 types of corporations that are involved in the healthcare field.

1. Listed corporations that own or manage healthcare facilities such as hospitals, nursing homes, surgical centers, community psychiatric facilities, sports medicine clinics and rehabilitation facilities. (examples: the Hospital Corporation of America, Bevely Enterprises) "most of these companies have performed spectacularly well for their investors, some have realized gains of up to 600 percent in the course of one year." (p.20)
2. Listed corporations that have purchased, bought out or otherwise acquired large medical partnerships. Wohl thinks this might be the most controversial ones, because the company basically "bought" the physicians

and because the profits end up "in the pockets" of the shareholders. The author wonders if this constitutes illegal professional fee-splitting. He clarifies: "Laws in many states…established rules…they deemed intermediate profiteering (that is, any second party profiting on a percentage basis from the practice of medicine and fee splitting) illegal. (p.21)(Example : Humana.) Some of those companies own medical facilities and professional medical personnel.

3. Listed corporations whose primary business is supplying goods and services to the health care field. Examples: Eli Lilly, Johnson and Johnson. "The pharmaceutical industry is expected to take in $150 billion in 1990." (p.21) "In recent years these suppliers have begun to take up the role of providers as well, e.g. care for elderly at home. (Upjohn joined Beverly Enterprises) or the president of Hospital Corporation of America also sits on the board of directors of Johnson & Johnson. "And the suppliers now have a strong say, an *interested* say in determining the utilization of the product they produce. The ethical and moral questions presented by such arrangement should be enough to fill a nation of prospective patients with considerable concern." (p.22)

4. Listed corporations whose primary business is elsewhere but which, over the last twenty years, have established subsidiaries in the health care field (Du Pont, Dow Chemical). They have a "vast capital …for acquisitional purposes." (p.22) Again, you see a blurring of supplier and provider function occurs with its concurrent problems.

5. Listed corporations that supply goods and services to a variety of markets but whose product account for large expenditures by the health care system. (IBM, Hewlett-Packard, General Electric, the nation's banking and insurance companies) "the high cost of their products and the profit potential they represent have interested others in doing so." (p.23)

6. Listed corporations that have sprung up in recent years to capture a specific field in the healthcare system (e.g. American Surgery Centers): Their concerns include genetic engineering, surgical practices and psychiatric services.

These six types of corporations (about 500) often are interrelated through common stock, board membership or joint ventures. They are liked by investors because they show tremendous growth in size and profit (p.24 ff) They are difficult to follow because they change their status constantly – like acquisitions and transferal of stock. Wohl calls it "a complicated maze of ownership and responsibility" (p.25)

For those of us who do not know much about the stock market, Wohl explains that there are groups of entities who can own stock: companies, institutions (like pension funds) and individuals. The system is regulated by the Securities and Exchange Commission (SEC), the Federal Trade Commission (FTC) and the Department of Justice. The FTC and the Department of Justice are supposed to watch out for possible violations, like conflict of interest, monopoly and fair-competition laws but they are, as the author feels, generally believed, to be poorly policed. (p.26) He feels that corporate ownership leads to "fewer and fewer hands serving on the board of more and more companies. The result is a cozy relationship of joint ownerships and common board members among …large firms". (p.27) So a corporation can own a health plan system, medical partnerships, insurance companies and hospitals. Take e.g. INA Health Plan Inc. INA management corporation owns shares of other companies like Humana or Beverly Enterprises. The author cites the example of Gerald D. Laubach, a director of Connecticut General, who was also the president of Pfizer Inc. (in 1984) Wohl writes "One looks in vain for some form of reaction from the …regulating agencies to this … activity" (p.27) He cites a takeover of a hospital by a corporation that resulted in an immediate increase of $50.00 per bed. He explains that with the government entering the healthcare – system, things began to change. It became the third party payer for the poor and elderly and it came with many regulations, programs and subsidies. (p.36) The doctors now had to send their bills to insurance companies or a government agency instead of to the individual patient. Also, a fourth entity became involved, the medical management company which, for a fee, kept the doctor's books and did the billing. (p.37ff) Cost for individual doctors became prohibitive and they began to form medical group. The physician began to feel more like an employee. At the same time hospitals began to act like businesses, too. Hospitals can be owned by universities, medical schools, the Veterans Administration or by a state, county, city or a municipal agency (or by doctors, health plans, religious orders, nonprofit endowment funds or by public or private corporations.) Wohl states: "in some cases, a university medical center attached to a private medical school may be owned by the state" (p.38 ff). Some hospitals are owned by a single entity, others can be part of a chain. The author points out that only the corporate chains distribute monetary gains to their shareholders.

As dealing with the financial aspects of hospitals became more complicated, administrators became the heads of hospitals, replacing doctors. Another problem was, that more and more people began to be covered through government or state programs but because the costs for these programs increased so quickly, the hospitals had problems to cover their costs. Many hospitals were forced to close and sell. The eager new buyers were the corporations.

Corporations wanted to employ doctors but these "incorporated" doctors had to use corporation owned buildings, labs, hospitals and refer their patients to other physicians belonging to the same corporation. (p.50)

Wohl points out that the low chance of creating a universal medical insurance, the generous Medicare and Medicaid payments, the financial problems of many hospitals, the employee mentality of many physicians and the aging of the population caused business to be interested. Health (and sickness) were "recession-proof". Medicine was a "high-cash-flow, low inventory, low investment affair." (p.53) Hospitals and healthcare is a large industry (in 1984 it amounted to 10% of the gross national product) ,(in 2022, 17.3 % according to the Centers for Medicare and Medicaid Services (CMS), a government entity. The Department of Health and Human Services is the largest bureaucracy in the world. (p.54) He writes: "no wonder that the corporate planners found the field inviting." He states: "A secure circle is formed when the goods of the suppliers (drugs, food, linens, X-rays, etc.) are assured a steady sale by the interested decisions of the provider". (p.54) "The suppliers now own shares in the hospitals that buy machines from them; they also own shares in the physician groups that prescribe the use of the machinery for their patients." (p.58) Wohl points out that shareholders expect growth. So companies are expected to buy more hospitals or to buy corporations that already own them. He continues: "the provider-supplier circle became even tighter when the corporations acquired the medical researchers, the most basic element of all."(p.66) Medical research used to be performed by academics in university hospitals and labs. (Some large pharmaceutical companies had their own labs.) Their work was paid by the government, i.e. the taxpayer. The researcher in a University would do his research and then publish the results in a scientific journal. His discovery belonged to the university. In the case of genetic engineering scientists sought additional private financial support. …soon entire companies were formed in order to support the work of two or three investigators." (p.67) There is litigation about the ownership of these discoveries. In these situations (where there is private business involved), it can happen that a scientist, rather than discussing the results with other scientists, can publicize his findings before that and cause the shares of that corporation to rise, even if his findings have problems.

Wohl writes that corporate business "now virtually encloses us in its provider – supplier grip from the moment of our birth until the final hour of life." (p. 71) (And the corporations won't let go of a good thing.)

David Armstrong wrote in 1995 (in Sociology of Health and Illness): "based on the surveillance of normal populations… this includes the problematization of normalcy." He says that everyone becomes a target. He uses the term "risk factor" and claims that any risk factor can point to a possible target. He writes: "Symptoms, signs, investigations and disease thereby become inflated into an infinite chain of risks. A headache may be a risk factor for high blood pressure, high blood pressure for a stroke. "A risk factor [is] any state of event from which a probability of illness can be calculated."

Wohl writes that the role of the physician has been greatly diminished and that federal and state governments underwrite 22% of the medical costs of the entire US-population and for 60% of people over 65. (taxpayers bear the cost of $ 1,8 trillion in healthcare cost in 2022, according to statnews.com on 12.19.23) The Center for Medicare and Medicaid (CMS) states that the Federal government and the State governments underwrote 409 billion for prescription drugs in 2022 and that the Federal government sponsors 33 % which is the largest share of total health spending. An American spends about $13, 500 on healthcare in 2022 (accord. To Peter G. Peterson foundation.)

Doctors don't have a say in the administration of healthcare services – it is run by professional administrators. He finds it astounding that "the profits gained from …medicine …show up in the pockets of stock market speculators." (p.87) He continues: "five hundred listed corporations have developed the infrastructure of a privately planned healthcare system that already owns a sizable percentage of both the acute beds and the chronic beds of the hospital facilities in this country and also supplies almost all the goods and materials to support the system."(p.87) He says that these corporations "capture" one-third of every healthcare dollar, they operate "outside the usual healthcare controlling mechanism." If they were independent there would be a healthy competition among them, but they are not: they are often interrelated, as mentioned above, by "common ownership of stock, shared board members …joint ventures and …transactions among themselves" (p. 87, 88) Wohl states: "The Medical Industrial Complex presents society with several moral and practical dilemmas, not the least of it is whether it should be allowed to exist at all." (p.96) "Corporations ['] …sole purpose is the creation of profits for their shareholders." But "in healthcare the highest quality care should be ensured." (p.96) He feels that doctors who work for or with a corporation deal with a "significant" conflict of interest. There are major ethical issues involved. The conflicts become clearer when you look at the relationship between drug companies and hospitals. When they are in the same hand (Johnsohn & Johnson owns a part of National Medical enterprises, Brystol-Myers owns part of the Hospital Corporation of America and Upjohn owns a piece of Beverly), the conflict of interest becomes very clear. The hospital prescribes the drugs that the partner-company produces, no matter if it's the best drug for a specific disease. So the patient may suffer in order for the corporation to make a profit.

Wohl concludes his book with "stating that widespread corporate involvement in healthcare is bad for us means that the wrong kind of people are exerting a great measure of control over the nation's health." (p.178). He warns of the real crisis looming:

> "It will occur if the U.S. mediglomerates achieve a monopoly position and completely take over American healthcare." (p.178)

and

> "The seeds of the problem have been planted in fertile corporate soil and only a strict ethical and legal control over the activities of the mediglomerates can ward off the collapse of the healthcare system that is otherwise sure to come." (p.180)

He feels that the danger of the medical monopoly is that they "control the system that is responsible for providing one of the fundamental rights of life-the best healthcare society can offer…corporations are only concerned with questions asked by their shareholders." (p.181)

Finally, Wohl believes that government, medical corporations and the medical profession should work together for the common good. He also feels that the public should become aware of the destructiveness of overutilization. Schools and colleges should teach about healthcare. Every American should turn into a prudent byer rather than being a wasteful spender. (p.192)

As we can see, Stanley Wohl showed us the danger of the involvement of healthcare corporations in our lives, but he is hopeful that a cooperation with doctors and the government might help to solve some of the problems.

I do not believe that this has happened, but to the contrary, that the corporations' influence has increased and is strengthened by their political influence as we will see in the following segments.

In her book "The Truth About the Drug Companies" (2004), the author Marcia Angell, M.D., former editor in chief of *The New England Journal of Medicine*, also examines the financial powers behind the pharmaceutical industry. Two laws were essential to increase these. (as mentioned before)

1. The Bayh-Dole Act was supposed to strengthen the position of American tech business globally.

> "[It] enabled universities and small businesses to patent discoveries emanating from research sponsored by the National Institutes of Health (NIH), the major distributor of tax dollars for medical research, and then to grant exclusive licenses to drug companies. Until then, taxpayer-financed discoveries were in the public domain, available to any company that wanted to use them. (p.7)

2.The Hatch-Waxmann Act expanded monopoly rights (patents) for brand-name drugs from eight to fourteen years by the FDA. (p. 10)

> Because of these two laws, Pharma became very wealthy and therefore very powerful. (In 2002 the profit from the 10

pharmaceutical companies listed in the Fortune 500 was higher than the profits from the other 490 businesses put together (35.9 billion vs. 33.7 billion. (p.11) The CEO of Bristol- Myers made almost 75 million and the same amount in stock options in 2001.(p.12)

The numbers Angell quotes almost seem quaint compared to newer numbers. In NY. Requirements.com (https://fortune.com/ranking/fortune500/2023/search) it is stated: (They list 30 companies, so that should compare to roughly 100 billion in the list quoted by Angell):

The worldwide pharmaceutical market in 2022 reached $1.4 trillion. (I only list the first 15 companies)

Pfizer earned:	$31.37 billion	($994,80 per second)
Johnson & Johnson:	$17.94 billion	
Merck:	$14.52 billion	
Roche:	$13.00 billion	
AbbVie	$11.84 billion	
BioN Tech	$10.34 billion	
Sanofi	$ 8.80 billion	
Novo Nordisk	$ 8.80 billion	
Moderna	$ 8.36 billion	
Novartis	$ 7.00 billion	
Amgen	$ 6.55 billion	
Bristol –Meyers Squibb	$ 6.33 billion	
Eli Lilly	$ 6.25 billion	
Abbott	$ 5.80 billion	
GSK	$ 5.30 billion	

In her introduction, Angell states:

> "Now primarily a marketing machine to sell drugs of dubious benefit,
> this industry uses its wealth and power to coopt every institution
> that might stand in its way, including the U.S. Congress, the Food and
> Drug Administration, academic medical centers and the medical
> profession itself." (p. XXVI)

By the way, R and D (research and development) are tax deductible and Angell claims that items that are considered under development are really promotional. (p.40) Considering the fact that at least a third of pharmaceuticals are licensed or acquired from outside sources. (p. 57) (If this doesn't seem fair to the American taxpayer, especially in view of the fact that he/she has to pay the highest prices for drugs it isn't.) (Angell calls it "paying twice." (p.65))

Angell writes that the NIH "has been friendly to big pharma as well. (…some senior scientists have had extensive financial dealings with drug companies.") (p.70)

Angell criticizes the "Me-too"drugs (or off-label) classified by the FDA as being no better than the drugs being already on the market to treat the same condition." (p.75). Companies just have to show the FDA that they are "effective", not "more effective", i.e. that they are better than nothing. Many are not better than older treatments. (p.75) "The FDA approves the drug not just for a particular use but for a specific dose."

As mentioned before, Angell criticizes pharma's manipulation of patent laws. She uses the example for Prozac. It was approved for depression in 1987, for obsessive compulsive disorder in 1994, for bulimia in 1996 and for geriatric depression in 1999. To avert the danger of termination of its patent, "it renamed Prozac Sarafem, colored it pink and lavender, and got FDA approval to market it for severe premenstrual symptoms. Same drug, same dose, but priced three times and a half times higher than generic Prozac at my local pharmacy." (p.83)

Angell lists three market conditions that have to exist to make a drug successful.

1. A market has to be large "to accommodate all the competing drugs." (p.83)

2. Its customers have to be able to pay. (Therefore no drug development for diseases that occur predominantly in poor countries)
3. The market has to be elastic "so it can expand." (p. 83-85)

She uses for an example the lowering of the definition of high blood pressure from 140 over 90 to 120 over 80. This added millions of customers for blood pressure drugs "despite the absence of convincing evidence of their benefit in this group." (p.85) Similar moves happened with cholesterol. The author states that diseases can be expanded or created. She claims that aging is now a disease and should – in the mind of the pharmaceutical industry - be treated. And that they promote (or create) diseases "to fit their drugs." "[Drugmakers] often expand the markets by coming up with slightly different uses and reap huge financial rewards...If a company tests a drug for a use slightly different from those of other drugs in the class, no other company can promote it for that purpose" (p.87). She claims that, in order to sell more drugs (like SSRI antidepressants) "they simply expanded the list of psychiatric disorders." She cites the bioethicist Carl Elliott:

> "The way to sell drugs is to sell psychiatric illness. It is in the interest of the pharmaceutical companies to broaden the category as far as possible and make the borders as fuzzy as possible." (p. 88)

She states "The fact that few psychiatric disorders have objective criteria for diagnosis makes these disorders easier to expand than most physical illnesses." (p.88) (She uses for an example "Social Anxiety Disorder")

Angell further asks the question about the reliability of trials and informs us that most clinical trials are sponsored by the drug manufacturers. "Drug companies now design clinical trials to be carried out by researchers... who are hired hands." (p.102.) "Sponsoring companies ...analyze and interpret the results and decide what, if anything, should be published." (p.102/103) Often researchers have financial ties to the pharmaceutical companies. (p.102,103)

Unfortunately, the NIH is not excluded from these ties. A journalist, David Willman from the Los Angeles Times "found that

> senior NIH scientists... routinely supplement their income by accepting large consulting fees and stock options from drug companies that have dealings with the institutes."

(The director of the institute, Harold Varmus, lifted the restrictions that had been established.) (p.104) Most senior scientists were not even required to file public disclosure of their outside income." (p. 106)

The Los Angeles Times stated in this regard:

> "Congress helped make this system and can help unmake it. Start with high-level hearings. Repeal the most destructive portions of the Bayh-Dole Act. Above all, restore the integrity of the National Institute of Health." (p.106)

As mentioned above, Angell is highly critical of the drug trials because of the connection between the researchers and the drug companies. She gives some examples, e.g. using young subjects to test a drug meant to be used for older people or manipulating doses to make a drug appear more effective than another one or incorrect administration of a drug or a trial being too short for medication that is supposed to be taken over a long time period, (taken over a long time period the product might be very harmful) or present only part of the results, namely the positive ones. She sees as the worst offense the suppression of negative results.

She continues:

> "when a drug company applies to the FDA for the approval of a new drug it is requires to submit the results of every trial it conducted...But it is not required to publish them." (p.111, 112)

Angell uses the example of the antidepressants Prozac, Paxil, Zoloft, Celexa, Serzone and Effexor and states that most clinical trials only last for six weeks. Results of trials often don't show much difference in the Hamilton Depression Scale. (Two point improvement on the sixty-two point Hamilton Depression Scale) (p. 113) when compared to a placebo showing no improvement. She continues:

> "More recently, there have been serious charges that manufacturers...have suppressed data indicating that the drugs are not only ineffective but sometimes dangerous in children." (p. 113) (s. see Lancet "Depressing research)

(In this regard, Linsey McGoey writes in her book "No such thing as a free gift":

"At the behest of the US Food and Drug Administration, GlaxoSmithKline, the manufacturer of <u>Paxil,</u> another bestselling SSRI, sent a letter to US physicians reporting that clinical trials testing Paxil had indicated a statistically significant, six-fold suicidal risk over placebo."(p.105))

Angell fears that the me-too (off-label) drugs are often pushed by companies who have a financial interest in them.That becomes obvious when you consider drug advertisements. They are only allowed in the US and New Zealand. Here the fear factor is used to motivate people to ask their doctor for certain prescriptions or they use stars in sports and movies to claim that certain medication helped them overcome their mental problem. The FDA has jurisdiction over prescription advertising and used to require full disclosure of the side effects. That changed in 1997:

"The FDA announced it would change the rules for broadcast ads. Instead of including a complete rundown of risks, companies would merely have to mention the major ones and refer viewers to a source of additional information." (p.123).

Ads are legally required to be sent to the FDA to be checked for "fair balance" (listing the risks and the benefits equally), but the FDA doesn't have enough reviewers and doesn't receive all the ads and under President Bush's administration their letters were sent out too late and not frequently enough. She feels that Americans are overmedicated with "all the side effects and drug interactions that go with it." She says:

"To stop drug companies from broadening their claims without evidence, they are not allowed to market drugs for "off-label" uses - that is uses not approved by the FDA. <u>Doctors, however, are not constrained by this law. They are permitted to prescribe drugs for whatever uses they want</u>. So if drug companies can somehow convince doctors to prescribe drugs for off-label uses, sales go up." (p. 137)

Drug companies try to circumvent this law by claiming that they just inform doctors about potential uses. They often sponsor pretense education and "flimsy" research and even give kickbacks. (although kickbacks are punishable by law.) Also continuing Medical Education is largely financed by drug companies or companies working for them. As Angell claims:"So here we have firms working for big pharma who are supposed to be providing impartial instruction about their clients' drugs."

Drug companies also woo "thought leaders". These are prominent experts in their field. She mentions the head of Brown University's Department of Psychiatry who made reportedly over $500,000 in one year consulting for drug companies that make antidepressants (p.143) As editor of the *New England Journal of Medicine* she required him and the professionals involved in a study of an antidepressant agent to list all their conflict- of interest disclosures. She found out that out of twelve principal authors only one did not have financial ties with BrystolMyersSqibb-which also sponsored the study and with many other psychoactive pharmaceutical agents. (even professional meetings like for Cardiology or Hematology are partly supported by pharmaceutical companies and their recommended pharmaceuticals are, in her opinion, not always the best remedy for a disease.) (p.144)
Angell warns against so-called advocacy groups:

> "Many of these groups are simply fronts for drug companies. People who suffer from a certain disease believe they have found a support network devoted to expanding awareness of the disease, but it is really a way for the drug companies to promote their drugs. Some people aren't even aware that a drug company is behind their advocacy groups; others believe the drug companies just want to help educate people…" (p.151, 152)

She writes:

> "One of the least savory marketing efforts is Wyeth's campaign to "educate" college students. What is really being marketed is the condition. If students can be convinced they have a treatable depression, selling the company drug Effexor is easy." (p.152)

Some colleges offer forums sponsored by these drug companies. Angell cites Alex Beam,a reporter for the BostonGlobe:

> "Millions of college students feel lousy, for any number of reasons: they are far from home; college is an unfamiliar and sometimes threatening environment; the object of their affection is inattentive. God knows we all have been there. Do they need a $120-a-month Effexor fix to see them through these tough years? Probably not. But who could be more susceptible, or vulnerable, than a boy or a girl making the transition to adulthood?" (p.153)

In her chapter "Marketing Masquerading as Research" Angell describes how a pharmaceutical company can turn a drug into a block buster. The first method is testing the drug for added conditions in clinical trials. If these are safe and effective, you can apply for FDA approval and market it for these additional uses.

The second way method: you can market the drug for unapproved ("off-label") uses-despite the fact that doing so is illegal... You do that by carrying out "research... that falls below the standard required for FDA approval, then "educating " doctors about any favorable results. That way, you could circumvent the law. You could say you were not marketing for unproved uses; you were merely disseminating the results of research to doctors-who can legally prescribe a drug for *any* use. (p.157)" She uses the case of the add on epilepsy drug Neurontin. One of their employees, David P. Franklin, charged the company who produced this drug, Pfizer, "had carried out a massive illegal scheme to promote Neurontin for off-label uses –mainly by paying academic experts to put their names on flimsy research papers that purported to show the drug worked for these other conditions" (p.157, 158) The makers of the drug wanted doctors to prescribe this drug for unapproved uses like pain and anxiety (more than a dozen uses!) . Neurontin became a blockbuster and made $2.7 billion in 2003. About 80% were for unapproved uses like bipolar disorder, post traumatic stress disorder, insomnia, restless leg syndrome, hot flashes, migraines and tension headaches "yet there is almost no good published evidence that it works for most of these conditions." (p.161)
(Today, Neurontin is also sold under its generic name Tiagabine and Gabapentin.)

As usual, it is being admitted by the drug industry that they don't know how the drug works, but on the medication guide (Revised 12/2020) the following information is given, approved by the FDA: Gabapentin can cause serious side effects like:

Thoughts or attempts to commit suicide

Depression

Anxiety

Agitation,

Panic attacks

Insomnia

Irritability

Aggressiveness

Violence

Jerky movements

Double vision

Unusual eye movements

Unexpected muscle pain

What happened to the unproven uses and the side effects? David Franklin was said to have cried when he saw that this medication was prescribed to children "off label" and what it did to them. Pfizer agreed to pay a fine of $430 million. (p. 161)

Angell describes the process a drug has to go through to get initial FDA approval:

> "Phase I through III clinical trials are directed toward getting initial FDA approval and they must meet the agency's scientific standards. Phase IV trials, in contrast, are studies of drugs already on the market (post marketing trials), and many of them don't have to meet any standard at all."

Angell writes that there are two legitimate reasons for Phase IV trials. First, to find out if the drug is effective for additional uses and to get FDA approval (must meet the same scientific standards as in Phase III trials.) Second, to find side effects that were missed in the earlier studies. (These studies were previously conducted in Europe before the drug was marketed in the US.) Now most drugs are first approved in the U.S. and they are given accelerated review by the FDA, which means that there may be less evidence that they work. The FDA requires drug companies to conduct Phase IV studies to ensure that the drug is safe. Angell claims that companies "drag their feet" to conduct these, because, of course, bad side effects are not good for business. She says: "As of 2003 only half of all the drugs that had undergone accelerated approval, had been fully investigated…" (p.163) She claims that the FDA can pull a drug from the market if the company does not do these studies, but, she claims, the FDA has never done this. She describes the form of the most common Phase IV trials (surveillance studies): The sponsor pays a doctor to puts a patient on a drug and the patients "answer a few simple questions how they fared. There is no randomization and no comparison group, so it's usually impossible to draw any reliable conclusion" (p.163). Angell has the suspicion that the drug companies contribute to these trials. She quotes a statement given by CenterWatch, a company that provides information about the clinical trial industry: "Sponsors must sometimes simplify study protocols to meet their marketing needs "(p.164)

The author informs us that there is a large increase in private contract research organizations that run trials for drug companies who use private doctors, many of whom, she feels, "essentially being paid to prescribe a company drug"(p.165) She feels that these Phase IV studies may be "totally unregulated",

> because the majority of them are never submitted to the FDA. They
> are mostly not published at all unless they show favorable results and
> are only published in "marginal journals."

She claims that now "huge advertising agencies own or employ research and education companies ." (p.166) So it's all about marketing.

In another chapter Angell criticizes the drug companies for their many attempts to increase the patent time in all kind of ways. One that I find particularly reprehensive is, after Congress approved the FDA's Modernization Act of 1997 adding six months of protection if the drug was tested on children. Because of this, many drug companies now test drugs for adults (like high blood pressure) (p.182) or Prozac (p.189) on children. I consider this almost to be child abuse because of the side effects the children may suffer.

Many times, a drug is used for another disease, often "created" for the drug. Angell uses the example of Prozac whose patent was running out. (s. a.) Lilly, the producer of the drug, renamed Prozac Sarafem and got the FDA to approve it for "premenstrual dysphonic disorder" (PMDD) (p. 189), a move, as she states, shows that diseases are created for drugs, not the reverse. Angell also names Paxil, an SSRI, me-too drug that is used for other conditions like "social anxiety disorder."

Probably the most important chapter in Angell's book is chapter 11 <u>"Buying influence – HOW THE INDUSTRY MAKES SURE IT GETS ITS WAY."</u> She describes that Medicare originally didn't pay for outpatient drugs when it was created in 1965, because drugs were not used as they are now. In 2003 <u>prescription drug benefit</u> was added to Medicare. Then Congress passed a bill that forbade bargaining for lower prices. Medicare who she thinks is the biggest purchaser of drugs has no influence on the prices.

She is afraid that the tremendous cost of the drugs will curtail other benefits and increase the price for seniors via deductions from their monthly checks and rising deductibles. Angell is not against Medicare prescription drug benefit but feels that drug prices should be negotiated between Medicare and the drug companies. She feels that all senior citizens should be covered for all cost - effective drugs. She asks the question why this seemingly can't be done and blames the lobbying industry on this and mentions Senator Durbin's (D- Ill) statement "…this lobby has a death grip on Congress "(p.196). Angell continues:

> "the industry is cozy with both Republicans and Democrats and with both the White House and Congress. But most of its attention is lavished on Republicans, and vice versa."

She cites a statement, reported in 1999 in the New York Times by John Nicholson, the chairman of the Republican National Committee, made to Charles A. Heimbold, then CEO of BristolMyersSquibb:

> "We must keep the lines of communication open if we want to continue passing legislation that will benefit your industry." (p. 197)

BristolMeyersSquibb ended up contributing $2 million to the Republican party in the year 2000, and asked their executives each to donate a thousand dollars to George W. Bush's campaign. (p.197) Angell continues:

<u>"In addition, big pharma contributes money to nearly every political campaign that may affect its fortune.</u> And recently the industry has put increasing sources into the formation and support in "ostensibly 'grassroot' organizations to promote its interests." (p. 198)

(According to <u>STATF</u> (www.statenews.com), an American health oriented website: <u>"More than two-thirds of Congress cashed a pharma campaign check in 2020"</u> <u>(June 9, 2021))</u>
 In the following, Angell examines the role of lobbyists more closely. (Her book, as mentioned, was written in 2004). She states that the pharmaceutical industry has by far the largest lobby in Washington. She claims:

> "in 2002 it employed 675 lobbyists (more than one for each member in Congress – at a cost of over \$91 million" (p.198)).

The list of lobbyist includes 26 former members of Congress and another 342 who had a connection with government officials. Some lobbyists were related to members of Congress like Scott Hatch, son of Senator Orrin Hatch and former Senator Birch Bay, father of Senator Evan Bay (D-Ind.) and also father of the "Bay-Dole Act." (p. 199) She continues:

> "In the 1999-2000 election cycle, drug companies gave \$20 million in direct campaign contributions plus \$65 million in "soft" money…The citizen group Common Cause … during the 1990… found …that Senator Hatch, Senator Bill Frist… Representative Bill Thomas…and Senator Joseph Lieberman, also enjoyed substantial industry favors." (p.200)

(According to the website "open secrets – following the money in politics") the drug companies and health product PACS gave \$ 13, 714, 885 in 2021/22.)

Angell examines the front groups "that masquerade as grass root organizations, e.g. Citizens for Medicare, who fought against any form of drug price regulation." Members of this "coalition" had ties to big pharma or United Senior Association. (p.202)

Angell writes:

"The influence of the pharmaceutical industry clearly reaches into the Bush Administration. Defense Secretary Donald Rumsfeld was CEO, president, and chairman of G.D. Searle …which … was bought by Pfizer. Mitchell E. Daniels, Jr., former White House budget director, was senior vice president of Eli Lilly. The first President Bush was on the Eli Lilly board of directors before becoming president." (p.202)

(In this regard, I want to cite parts of an article published by the Psychiatric Services APA (<u>American Psychiatric Association</u>) online, written by Michael F. Hogan, PHD. on Nov.1, 2003:

"On April 29, 2002… George W. Bush announced <u>The President's New Freedom Commission on Mental Health.</u> He said "We need a healthcare system which treats mental illness as the same urgency as physical illness." He announced the creation of a mental health commission. Its goals were: "early screening, assessment and treatment…this must become a national goal." The members state "prevention is best" and "schools are in a key position to identify mental health problems and provide appropriate services -or links to services." They suggest an annual mental health check-up ("-with assurance of parental consent") Their final recommendation is to screen for mental health disorders in primary care settings and to use TEENSCREEN as a model. (TEENSCREEN is part of the Foundation for Suicide Prevention. It was terminated in 2012. <u>Wikipedia</u> (accessed on May 9, 2024) writes the following about TEENSCREEN:
"There is opposition to mental health screening programs in general and TEENSCREEN in particular, from civil liberties, parental right and politically conservative groups. Much of the opposition is led by groups who claim that the organization is funded by the pharmaceutical industry. Parents had filed a law-suit claiming the screening was done without parents' permission. It was developed by David Shaffer who is known for his connection to the pharmaceutical industry.)

<u>The Medical Whistleblower Advocacy network</u> (http://medicalwhistleblower .org>teenscreen) writes under the title: New Freedom Commission and TEENSCREEN:

"The commission… recommended screening…children for emotional disturbances in order to increase the use of highly controversial and inadequately tested pharmaceutical drugs. Many of these drugs were found to be dangerous and had serious long term health effects as well as being physically addictive that it was almost impossible to take the patient off them. <u>There are few potential benefits …except increased profits for the pharmaceutical companies</u>. There are serious concerns about the potential for unnecessarily causing neurological damage…Through the guise of TMAP (Texas Medication Algorism Project) (it began as an alliance of individuals from the University of Texas, the pharmaceutical industry and the Mental Health and Correction Systems of Texas) <u>…critics contend that the drug industry has methodically influenced the decision making of elected and appointed public officials to gain access to citizens in prisons and State psychiatric hospitals.</u>"

"Allen Jones was the investigator for the Office of Inspector General regarding the approval of psychotropic drugs by the Food and Drug Administration. Allen Jones was a former investigator in the Commonwealth of Pennsylvania Office of Inspector General (OIG) Bureau of Special Investigations. His very detailed report can be found on the <u>Psychrights.org website</u>." Jones stated that behind the recommendations of the New Freedom Commission was the "political/pharmaceutical alliance." It was this alliance, according to Jones, which developed the Texas project, specifically to promote the use of newer, more expensive antipsychotics and antidepressants. He further claimed this alliance was "poised to consolidate the TMAP effort into a comprehensive national policy to treat mental illness with expensive, patented medications of questionable benefit and deadly side effects , and to force private insurers to pick up more of the tab.")
But back to Angell.

She lists some of the favors drug companies have gotten from Congress, like extension for drug monopolies, tax breaks, prohibition of importing prescription drugs from other countries even if manufactured in the US. (Only the manufacturers are allowed to do this.) She continues:

"Other congressional actions target the FDA's ability to regulate the industry. The 1997 Food and Drug Administration Modernization Act, for instance, was a giant giveaway to the pharmaceutical industry... It required the agency to lower its standard for approving drugs... it has not authorized the FDA to require that new drug to be tested against older ones as a condition of approval. The fact that drug companies get away with comparing drugs only with placebos is what makes it possible for the industry to live on me-too drugs...One of the least known but biggest gifts Congress gave Big Pharma was to authorize an <u>industry –supported private company to decide whether Medicaid</u> would pay for off-label uses of prescription drugs. As mentioned before, while drug companies are not permitted to market drugs for uses not approved by the FDA, doctors may prescribe drugs for whatever reason they like. That leaves open the question of whether insurers will pay – not a small matter since <u>as many as half of all</u> prescriptions are written for off-label uses. This question is particular important for Medicaid which is the largest government program that pays for outpatient drugs. In 1997, Congress named <u>Drugdex</u> Information Service as one of the three organizations that would decide which off-label uses Medicaid would cover...If a use is listed there, Medicare must pay for the drug when it is prescribed for that use." (p.203, 204) (There are, additionally, two other federally recognized directories both of which are nonprofit).

She continues:

"in 2003, according to the Wall Street Journal, Drugdex listed 203 off-label uses for the top-selling drugs in the United States. They included ...48 off label uses for Neurontin, the epilepsy drug. According to the company, Neurontin can be used for hiccups, nicotine withdrawal, migraine ...and Medicare has to pay for it. Because Drugdex lists so many more off-label uses than the other directories, it in effect sets the standard. It cites articles to support its listings, but the articles are not required to meet any scientific criteria...<u>So here is a company with close ties to the pharmaceutical industry that singlehandedly determines coverage for about half of all prescriptions written for Medicaid recipients. And all at taxpayer expense...this arrangement bypasses FDA approval...</u>"(p.205, 206)

Angell writes:

> "Congress also put the FDA on the pharmaceutical industry's payroll. In 1992, it enacted the <u>Prescription Drug User Fee Act</u> which authorized drug companies to pay user fees to the FDA. These were to be employed to expedite approval of drugs. Fees originally amounted to $310.000 per new drug application, and soon accounted for about half the budget of the agency's drug evaluation center. That makes the agency dependent on an industry it regulates. "(p.208)

In 2002 the fee was increased to $567.000 per new drug application. User fees altogether account for $260 million a year. (in 2005). Angell states:

> "The lion's share is still earmarked to speed drug approval. (p.208)… <u>industry employees constitute more than half of the FDA staff involved in approving drugs.</u> (source cited on p.209) Yet, the faster the approval process, the more likely it is that dangerous drugs will reach the market. Indeed, over the decade since the Prescription Drug Use Fee Act was enacted, a record <u>thirteen prescription drugs have had to be withdrawn from the market-after they caused hundreds of deaths."</u> (source cited on p. 209).

The approval process, she claims is much slower in other countries. Also, the FDA is much slower taking dangerous drug off the market than other countries. She names the diabetes drug Rezulin. It was taken off the market in Britain in 1997 because it caused liver failure in 1997 but it was not removed from the market in the US two and half a year later "after it had caused at least sixty three deaths." (p.209) Angell also explains that the FDA has eighteen standing advisory committees on drug approval. "Many members of these committees have financial connections to interested companies." (p.210)
She further states that one of the biggest strains on state budgets is Medicare "and the fastest growing component of that is prescription drug spending" (p.227)

Finally, Angell urges the population to ask their senators and representatives if they receive campaign contributions and the amount or sources of income.

In this regard, let me cite <u>Richard Belzer and David Wayne</u> who quote Jack Law in their book "Corporate Conspiracies" (2017):

> "The drug business is the most profitable in the entire world of capitalism." (p. 118 (Jack Law's "Big pharma: Exposing the global Healthcare agenda" (New York: Carrol and Graf, 2006))

Let's first examine their growing power. One of the world's leading health writers with many awards, including Harvard's Harkness Fellowship, <u>Ray Moynihan</u>, and <u>Alan Cassels</u>, a pharmaceutical policy researcher at the University of Victoria, British Columbia, have written a book "<u>Selling sickness</u> – How the world's biggest Pharmaceutical companies are turning us all into patients" (2005.)

They begin by quoting a Merck executive who said it was his dream to make drugs for healthy people. The authors feel that his dream has become true:

> "The ups and downs of daily life have become mental disorders, common complaints are transformed into frightening conditions, and more and more people are turned into patients. With promotional campaigns that exploit our deepest fears of death, decay and disease, the <u>$500 billion pharmaceutical industry</u> (in 2005!) (worldwide 1.6 trillion in 2023 according to the website "Statista") is literally changing what is means to be human…Mild problems are painted as serious disease, so shyness becomes a sign of social anxiety disorder and premenstrual tension a mental illness called premenstrual dysphoric disorder. Everyday sexual difficulties are seen as sexual dysfunctions …distracted office workers now have adult ADD. Just being "at risk" of an illness has become a "disease." (p.X.)

The authors feel that relatively healthy people are thus exposed to unnecessary high expenses and "the very real danger of sometimes deadly side effects." (p. X) They state that

> <u>America has "less than 5% of the world's population "but consumes" almost 50% of the global market in prescription drugs." (p.XI)</u>

The most promoted categories are heart medication and antidepressants. The authors describe how an advertising executive, Vince Parry, helps companies to change or emphasize old diseases or create new ones. (p.XI) Drug companies, advertisement executives and medical expert get together to create a disease. (s. Parry "The art of branding condition" Medical Marketing and Media(MM&M), May 2003, pp.43 -9) This will bring "billions in soaring drug sales" (The authors cite J. Coe in "The lifestyle drugs outlook to 2008": "The coming years will bear greater witness to the corporate sponsored creation of disease." (p.XII)

The authors point out that the marketing executives don't write the rules for diagnosing illnesses, but they "underwrite those who do." (p.XIII) by sponsoring medical meetings. In some cases, medical experts take money from the drug companies. Often, senior specialists are on their payroll and they are drawing the "boundaries of the diseases wider and wider while ...the causes ...are portrayed as narrowly as possible" (p.XIV) like reducing heart problems to high blood pressure or high cholesterol.

They state that the motive behind the sale of drugs is the "marketing of fear." They use as an example parents' fear of teenage suicide to sell powerful drugs. Often, they state, the medication causes the harm that they are supposed to prevent.

Drug companies have become very profitable, but at a high cost for insurers and the government, i.e. the taxpayer. The authors wish that the public recognizes the dangers, will discuss them and will come to a better solution.

In the following the book describes several diseases and the selling of drugs to treat them. They begin with high cholesterol and the huge profits made with medication for it. They cite a researcher who feels that cholesterol lowering drugs (statins) have a place in medicine, but that there are many ways to benefit your health like diet and exercise. One drug, Lipitor, was a huge moneymaker (more than $10 billion) for its creator, Pfizer. The number of people defined as having high cholesterol has grown "astronomically." These guidelines are regularly revised. In 2001 a new panel of experts lowered the "dangerous" level and thus increased the pool of "patients" from thirteen million (in the 1990s) to 36 million. The chair of the panel who decided this (and five of the fourteen members) had financial ties to statin manufacturers. In 2004 these guidelines were updated again. Now 40 million Americans "could benefit by taking the drug." Eight of the nine experts who wrote the latest guidelines were on the payroll of the major drug companies. (Sources cited on p.3 and 4). "It is estimated that

> almost 90 percent of those who write guidelines for their peers have conflicts of interest because of financial ties to the pharmaceutical industry" (source cited on p.4)

Another concern is the industry's influence over doctors. Continuing medical education for doctors is close to half funded by drug companies, scientific research is close to 60 percent funded by them and testing for drugs for depression is close to 100 percent.

> "Almost all the clinical trials of the new antidepressants were funded by their manufacturers rather than public or not-for-profit sources." (source cited on p. 6)

 These are discussed and evaluated by yearly meetings sponsored by the industry and "often hosted by medical societies like the American Heart Association, themselves partially underwritten by drug companies." (source cited on p.6). The senior physicians who write the guidelines, conduct research, educate their colleagues and publish papers, might be employed at prestigious academic schools or might be working for drug companies as advisers and speakers. (p.6). The authors use the example of Dr. Bryan Brewer, a senior official who works for the publicly funded National Institutes of Health (NIH). At a meeting of the American Heart Association he described the statin Crestor (AstraZeneca) as safe and effective. It turned out that he had received two hundred thousand dollars from outside sources, including from drug companies. (source cited on p.6 and 7.)

The authors see as a fundamental danger that doctors not only are "helping to sell the medicines, but helping to sell a particular definition of disease that expands markets for those medicines." (p.7). The authors are using the example of high blood pressure. They claim that in order to sell more medication the threshold for the ailment has been downgraded (more than 40 million are defined as having this disease) (I have a couple of friends who had initially high blood pressure and diabetes, lost weight and don't have these diseases any longer, but were told to stay on their medication. Both friends are, by the way, on Medicare!) If you familiarize yourself with the side effects of statins you realize that there are dangerous side effects connected to these medications. (although the authors state that these drugs are beneficial if you already have heart problems.)

One dangerous development is the creation of astroturfing , "the creation of fake grassroots campaigns by public relations professionals in the pay of large corporations." (p.9) (s, Angell) (I recently read an interview with a famous actress who claimed that she had been depressed but that she is doing so much better because she is taking Zoloft.- It was not revealed who paid for her statement)

The authors cite "a gobal survey from Britain estimated that <u>two-thirds of all patient advocacy groups and health charities now rely on funding from drug companies or</u> <u>device manufacturers.</u>" (p.10) Johnson & Johnson and Pfizer contribute the most. Of course, advertising contributes greatly to selling diseases that might not be real diseases and the drugs to treat them. (The World Health Organization (WHO) was concerned about the inaccurate description of the medication and urged "he health authorities to be more vigorous in regulating pharmaceutical promotion..." (cited on p.15)) On the contrary, they state, that U.S. government backed guidelines recommend "that the entire population over twenty years old-around 200 million people- should have their blood cholesterol levels regularly tested." (cited on p.16)

After Cholesterol the authors direct their attention to <u>depression</u>. They state that mental health specialists claim that the disease is most likely due to a chemical imbalance in the brain. (I checked and saw that the NIH actually states that it <u>is thought </u>to be caused by a chemical imbalance. "It is thought" is such a slippery phrase. If it turns out that it isn't true, nobody can claim that you lied.) Nobody has ever been able to prove this or to measure this. I have talked about the medications for this in a separate chapter. They are big money makers <u>($20 billion)</u> (p.23) The authors state that the benefits are much more modest and the risks far greater than generally assumed. The clinical trials have almost all been funded by the manufacturers and the side effects like a decrease in sexual interest, severe withdrawal symptoms, risks of suicide in the young, is downplayed. Amazingly, it is the very fear of suicide of the young that has people turn to these medications. (sources cited on p. 24). Dr. Marcia Angell (s. a.) found that only a few psychiatrists had no ties to the pharmaceutical industry. (cited on p. 26) The authors cite psychiatrist Dr. <u>Loren Mosher</u> who claims

They quote another psychiatrist, David Healy, who feels "that the serotonin theory has been overplayed in order to help sell the selective serotonin reuptake inhibitor drugs including Prozac, Paxil and Zoloft." (p.28) The authors further doubt the claim that 30 percent of Americans have a mental disorder. The original research whose lead researcher was Dr. Ron Kessler, was challenged by psychiatrist Dr. William Narrow, who was working at the time for the NIH, the government funded National Institute of Health. He found the serious cases of mental disorders to be significantly lower. (p. 29) He saw that many people with mild problems had been included in the survey. But Kessler insists "Let's treat them" (cited on p.30). The authors continue:

> "he has taken funds from several companies… most recently from Lilly, GSK (GlaxoSmithKline) and Pfizer —the makers of the world's three top-selling antidepressants" (source cited on p.30).

Kessler's survey included fourteen different countries and resulted in widely different numbers. The authors conclude that the survey included very mild cases that needed no treatment and criticize the term "unmet need" that is used to push aggressive drug marketing. (p.31). The authors cite Australia where general practitioners attended an educational program about depression that was partly funded by a drug company. Antidepressant prescriptions tripled and rates among the fifteen to twenty-four year olds increased tenfold. (sources cited on p. 32). The screening test of this program (funded by BristolMyersSquibb) was so broad that it classified 49 percent as having a "mental disorder" (p. 32). Later, the researchers from the Monash Medical Centre in Melbourne examined the test and found that most of the tested people were not disordered. The authors cite the researchers "Labeling a significant number of people who are not depressed as "probably depressed" might reasonably considered harm. We do not want to replace… under-recognition with over-recognition…"(p. 33) The authors point out the dangerous side effects of antidepressants. Serzone was withdrawn from the market because it was linked to hepatitis and liver failure in some patients.

Prozac, Paxil and Zoloft can cause serious sexual difficulties, serious problems with withdrawal, but most serious is the side effect of suicidal behavior and thinking in children and adolescents that was revealed when the public demanded to see the drug company funded trials. The "industry –friendly FDA "had to get involved. There were two public meetings that examined this problem." The first one took place in February 2004 in Bethesda, Maryland. A witness, Tom Woodward, described an incident concerning his daughter. A top student, she had been diagnosed with depression (the parents described it as a "normal bout of teenage trouble") and been prescribed Zoloft. A week after beginning to take the drug she hung herself. (cited on p.34). There were many similar testimonies before this hearing. Professor Mark Hudak from the University of Florida "urged the FDA to take action" (p.35) He felt that children with minor problems are "put on these drugs with terrible consequences." (cited on p.35). The regulators suggested that the use of these drugs *increased* suicidal behavior from 2 percent to 4 percent. (p.35). Also, the clinical trials showed that these drugs (except Prozac) did not work better than placebos. Britain tried to stop the presciption to children. US authorities tried to get the FDA to add a black box warning to antidepressant labels (cited on p.35). A huge problem with the FDA is "That the FDA relies on industry funds for much of its drug review work." (p.36) Remember, the FDA is supported by our tax money, but is dependent on corporations whose main purpose is to make money. The group "Public Citizen" was trying to change this situation, but lost the fight.)

Tom Woodward who has lost his daughter so tragically, has become an activist and he sees the "pharmaceutical industry's unhealthy influence over the U.S. Congress and the White House. He is a campaigner for much tougher and more independent drug regulation." (p.36)

The authors quote the London general practitioner Dr. Lona Heath: "many ordinary life experiences get a label and a drug."(p.36) She also feels that the screening checklist is too broad, like have you been "down in the dumps" (p.36) as a category.

Another "mental illness" the authors examine is "Social anxiety disorder." They describe the case of a young woman, Deborah Olguin, who had had problems doing well on job interviews. She saw a commercial for Paxil and decided to take the medication. (They cite one of the team of a large PR company who said "We're not only tapped in the latest trend, we set them.") (cited on p.120)). So "shyness and uneasiness in social situations" became a mental disease. Paxil is <u>worth $3 billion</u> a year and became the world's top selling antidepressant. (p.120) They often cultivate "the marketplace prior to approval."(by the FDA) (source cited on p.121) The drug company GSK's (GlaxoSmithKline) goal was to show that Social Anxiety Disorder was a severe condition . There were two objectives: "to generate extensive media coverage" about the "disorder" and to surpass Zoloft in sales (Prozac was no.1). The medical and advocacy groups Social Anxiety Coalition were sponsored by drug companies. (cited on p. 122) The drug trials were run by Dr. Murray Stein. He has been a paid consultant to seventeen drug companies, including GSK. Paxil was approved by the FDA in 1999. (sources cited on p.123). Deborah Olguin still took Paxil five years after beginning the drug, because she experienced horrible withdrawal symptoms. Because it is so expensive she drives to Mexico to buy the drug. She has never been warned that there is a suggestion of an increase in suicidal thinking and behavior in children and adolescents (which caused the British health authorities to ban the drug for them.) (p.124)

Vince Parry feels that anxiety and mood disorders have "been ripe for 'condition branding'." He explains that there is no blood test for these condition, so psychiatrists have to rely on a checklist of symptoms for Social Anxiety Disorder. He cites one symptom [it is a]"general feeling of uneasiness among other individuals that might limit your ability to participate" (p. 127) Critics feel that there is a blurring between normal life and disease, that "common shyness seem like a mental disease" (p.130) "Thousands of others, like Deborah Olgium, are taking legal action against the company (with the help of the law firm Baum Hedlund in Los Angeles), alleging they were not warned of the drug's potential to cause withdrawal and dependence." (p.132-133) The author cite psychiatrist Professor David Healy, an expert advisor for Baum Hedlund. Healy was especially concerned with the aspect of suicidal behavior in relation to <u>Paxil.</u> As an expert in the legal case, he got access to GSKs files and discovered that

> the company was very well aware of the fact that the drug caused an increase in suicidal thinking and behavior. Medical authorities who

looked into this problem also found out that other antidepressants show similar dangers. (p.134.)

They found also, that "there was no good evidence that the antidepressants were any better than a placebo." (p.134) Despite these facts, the consume of antidepressants increased dramatically. The FDA finally required a black box warning for all antidepressants. (p.134-135) In 2004, New York attorney Elliot Spitzer sued GSK, accusing them of misleading the public about the ineffectiveness and danger of the drug. GSK rejected the charges as unfounded, but paid $2.5 million to avoid further action by the court. "yet, according to press reports, an internal GSK memo sent to its drug detailers in 2003 specifically advises [them] not to discuss the potential link with suicidal behavior with prescribing doctors" (p.135) There is a global move to make trials accessible to the public. "that may bring a long overdue transparency to industry funded medical science." (p.135)

In the epilogue of their book titled "What can we do?" the authors recommend the use of a new journal "PLOS medicine" (Public Library of Science (plos.org) which provides free access to all of its scientific articles. The journal won't accept drug companies' advertisements or company-funded studies "considered dressed up as science." (p.196) The authors warn: "Challenging and questioning the status quo is the first step for anyone concerned about the selling of sickness" (p.197). They think it is very helpful to discuss with friends and family if an apparent problem is really a disease "or simply one of the ups and downs of ordinary life". (p.197) There are sources that are wholly independent of drug companies like the ECRI (Emergency Care Research Institute (https://home.ecri.org) in the U.S. or the International Cochrane Collaboration or the American Medical Student Association. (p.198)

The researchers at NYRequirements.com used CorporateWatch.org to answer their question why these companies made so much money and they found several reasons:

- They concentrate on the most profitable drugs that treat common chronic diseases because the demand will always be high. (They had neglected vaccines until Covid-19 with heavy government support appeared.)

- They rely on patents to avoid competition, thus create monopolies and set high prices. (The patents are valid for twenty years after their invention which means that the prices can stay high. (s. Angell) (The authors cite Humira, an immunosuppressive drug for autoimmune diseases like arthritis or Crohn's disease. It can cost up to $8,000 for a supply for two weeks.)
- There is a massive profit margin. The drug companies spend about 20% of their sales revenue on R and D. (Research and Development). Once on the market, they are cheap to produce. The authors use for an example insulin that costs about $6 to produce but sells for $275 in the U.S. The gross profit margin of pharmaceutical companies in the U.S. was 71%.
- There is minimal risk involved. Most of the research on new drugs is done in Universities, government labs and smaller research companies. Much of it is funded by the government. The National Institute of Health (NIH) a government institution, gives about $40 billion a year to Universities, medical schools and other research organizations. Then the big pharmaceutical companies acquire a license for these drugs. (So the taxpayer pays twice, once for the research and again for the drug, often through Medicare or Medicaid) (s. Angell)
- The employment of lobbying. (The main U.S. lobby group is Pharmaceutical Research and Manufacturers of America (PHRMA)) Pharma spends more on lobbying than any other industry, almost double of the runner-up, the insurance industry. In 2022 the pharmaceutical industry spent more than $372 million on federal lobbying (according to OpenSecrets.org) They have more than 1,450 lobbyists, 66% of whom are former government employees. The U.S. also has the highest drug prices in the world. "Coincidence?" asks the author of this article, Julia Tortorice, wo posted it. She points out that drugs save many lives but that many people who need drugs can't afford them.

(Investopedia states naively: "In the United States, antitrust legislation is in place to restrict monopolies, ensuring that one business cannot control a market and use that control to exploit its customers.")

Melody Petersen, a highly acclaimed investigative reporter, severely criticizes the drug companies in her book "Our daily meds" (2008). She says (s. Angell):

"The drug companies' chain of influence is so complete that there are few people left to look objectively at the effects of their products on the nation's health or the consequences of their power for society. <u>Washington is the axis of the industry's power. The pharmaceutical companies spent more on lobbying between 1998 and 2004 than any other industry. By 2004 ... there were more than two [lobbyists] for each member of Congress -They use their wealth to buy influence.</u>" (p.10)

The US is the only country in the world that does not control prescription drug prices. "In too many cases, whether a medicine helps or harms a patient has become secondary to how much it will bring shareholders its profit." (p. 11) "None is suited better for condition branding ...than the field of anxiety and depression." (p. 22), because mental disorders are rarely based on measurable physical symptoms. "Many of the growing numbers of psychiatric conditions listed in the Diagnostic and Statistical Manual of mental disorders were brought to light through funding by the pharmaceutical companies. For instance, Premenstrual Dysphoric Disorder (PMDD) was created. Marketing for this was not successful in Europe. European regulators forced Lilly to stop selling Prozac for it, saying it was not a well - established disease. (p.23)

According to the author, the pharmaceutical companies wanted to "create enthusiasm among the public for lifelong medication use which they called compliance 2005." (p.63). "A two- day conference for industry executives in November 2005 was devoted solely to techniques used to keep people complying with their prescription schedule. Consultants estimated the drug makers could add billions of dollars to their annual sales if they could keep people taking their meds."(p.63)   A step in this direction was the collection of personal and medical information on every American. "A firm named <u>PharMetrics</u> (s. chapter 25) said in 2005 that it had the complete set of pharmacy and medical claims of more than fifty-five million Americans, obtained from insurance companies, pharmacies and other medical providers. Marketers also created websites to attract people looking for health information.

The author presents some information on <u>"National Depression Screening Day"</u> (under notes no.55, p.351). It was created by Dr. Douglas Jacobs, "consultant to at least one pharmaceutical company. The group tested more than two hundred thousand Americans for mental illness each year…<u>the screenings</u> <u>were funded by</u> <u>five drug companies, all sellers of antidepressants</u>… In 2004 a panel of experts brought together by the federal government warned that there was a lack of evidence that such screenings decreased suicide attempts or actually helped people more than hurt them."(p.351, no.55) The author describes a case that involved the drug <u>Neurontin.</u> (s. Angell) Doctors were paid to prescribe this drug in doses that were double of what the FDA recommended which aggravated the children's behavior. They threw tantrums and became aggressive. There were many other incidents that showed how damaging the drug was. One employee, David P. Franklin, (s. a.) of the pharmaceutical company that produced the drug, contacted a law firm which used the <u>False Claim Act</u> (A federal law passed in 1863 under Lincoln to protect the army against the fraudulent war profiteers) to pursue this case (p.244) The public didn't find out until the government had time to investigate and decided if it wanted to join the lawsuit. (p.245) The producer of the drug was finally convicted and had to pay $430 million. (p.245) The author states that the Neurontin case "was hardly an aberration in the pharmaceutical industry.

> In 2005, an official in the U.S. Justice Department testified before
> Congress that <u>the government had begun 180 separate investigations</u>
> <u>of the marketing practices of pharmaceutical companies. The</u>
> <u>investigations involved dozens of companies and hundreds of drugs."</u>
> (p.249)

A reporter took a closer look at <u>Ritalin</u> and found out that two thirds of daycare centers surveyed in Eastern Iowa reported that they distributed medicine for ADD to their young attendees. (p.85). Researchers from Iowa State University found out (in the 1990) that 25 % of the students took Ritalin. Petersen found out that the school had formed a partnership with a local mental health group. She continues: "Wellmark, the insurer, had helped spur the rise in antidepressants by asking physicians in its network to have patients…answer nine written questions about their mood…the questionnaire allowed primary care doctors to swiftly diagnose depression and prescribe an antidepressant." (p. 92) The questionnaire was known by the name of <u>Prime-MD and was created by Pfizer</u>, as Kirk and Kutchins had pointed out. (s. a.) Petersen recalls her visit to a pediatrician in Iowa who told her that many of the children she treated were on several prescription stimulants and that there almost were no studies that follow what happens to these children. (p.94) What concerned the doctor the most is that "children who need help so desperately almost always receive it in a chemical form." (p. 94) The author states that the use of Ritalin, Adderall or Concerta increased sharply in the early 1990s "as the pharmaceutical companies increased their promotion and

> after federal lawmakers made attention deficit disorder a protected
> disability under the Individuals with Disabilities Education Act.
> Lawmakers also agreed that families could collect federal disability
> payments known as supplemental security income(SSI), in cases in
> which children were impaired by the disorder." (p.97)

 She continues:" Doctors wrote almost five times as many prescriptions for Ritalin and similar drugs in1996 as they had just six years before. By 2004 2.5 million American children were taking these drugs, including almost 10 percent of all ten-year-old-boys." (p.97) Petersen continues: Some critics "say ...that normal childhood behaviors are now considered symptoms of mental illness" (p.98) and points out, like many mental health specialists that there are no blood tests or other ways to test physically for attention deficit disorder or any other mental illnesses " (p.98).
She quotes Dr. Stewart A. Kirk: (s. a.) who said :

> "American psychiatrists and drug companies... are eying the
> lengthening list of disorders in the DSM "like a lumber company
> lusting after a redwood forest."" (p.99)

The author further describes how in 2005 Iowa schoolboard members heard presentations about a program named TeenScreen initiated by the Columbia university professor of psychiatry, Dr. David Shaffer, who has worked as a consultant for some of the big pharmaceutical companies. (s.a.) His team reported in 1996 that nearly 21 % of American children had a mental disorder. The staff offered to test school children on a regular basis for mental health problems, ostensibly to prevent suicides. She points out that scientific studies could not prove that such screening outweighed the possible harm that could be done by prescribing medication to students who are not mentally ill. In the year

2000 Dr. Shaffer announced that he had shown that screening adolescents at school could find those at risk for suicide. <u>Solvay Pharmaceuticals, the makers of Luvox, gave checks, totalling $500,000 to the Foundation for Suicide Preventionn</u> whose president Dr. Shaffer was. In 2005 the founders chair was a former chief executive of Solvay and executives from Pfizer and Johnson and Johnson. (p.101). "By the end of 2005 at least seven school districts in Iowa were using TeenScreen." (p. 101, 102)

> "Some of the antidepressant drug manufacturer had also pushed in recent years to screen Iowa children who were much younger. For example, Pfizer, GlaxoSmithKline and Eli Lilly paid in 2001 to promote health screening for all kids during what organizers called <u>Child Health Month.</u> The event's main message was that one out of every five Iowa children had a mental illness that could be diagnosed and treated….Iowa governor Tom Vilsack, the University of Iowa and the state's pediatricians urged the parents to have their children tested." (p.102)

The author points out that the FDA signed on June 15th, 1938, into law that required companies to test the safety of medicines before they are sold. The federal government does not require drug companies to prove that a new drug is better than those on the market. (s.Angell) She claims that most drugs are only tested on a few thousand people and just for a few weeks.

Petersen remarks how often companies keep negative results of their tests secret (s.a.) and cause much harm by doing this. She uses the example of <u>Paxil</u> (s. a.), whose manufacturers had kept studies that it had conducted to test its effectiveness on teenagers secret. The studies showed that the drug did not ease the children's depression, but increased doubly suicidal thinking in children who took the drug compared to those who used a placebo. (p.204) (s. a.) The author continues:

> "No one knows how many pharmaceutical studies have been kept secret after they showed a drug did not work or cause harm. Numerous reviews have found that <u>at least 50% of pharmaceutical trials have never been published.</u> The percentage may be far higher. One group of reviewers looked at clinical trials for pain medicine

known as non-steroidal anti-inflammatory drugs or NSAIDs. Their analysis found that only one of thirty-seven experiments involving the pain medicines had been published. "GlaxoSmith Kline settled the lawsuit brought by Spitzer by promising to begin disclosing the results of all its clinical trials to the public." (p. 205)

In 2007 Congress required the government to keep a list of drug trials. The author states that many studies remain "in boxes in the dark corners of empty warehouses." (p.205) She describes faulty trials involving Ritalin. Novartis, the maker of the drug had, for instance, removed children whose behavior had not improved or who became sick from the results.

"In 2005 researchers at Oregon Health & Science University set out to evaluate the scientific evidence that had been published on the medicines prescribed for attention deficit disorders." (p.208). <u>They found that "there was no good scientific evidence that Ritalin or any of the other drugs were safe for treating children for longer than six months." (p.211)</u>

The author points out that federal law forbids companies from promoting medicines for uses that the government has not approved. (s. Angell) "To gain approval they must show evidence of the drug's effectiveness by performing "adequate and well –controlled investigations."(p.224) Rules are different for doctors. "Once a medicine is approved, it is legal for physicians to prescribe it in any way that they believe is best for their patient. They do not need government approval, for instance, to prescribe an antiseizure medication for a child diagnosed with ADD" (p.224) This is called "Off label". Often patients do not know that they are given an off-label prescription.

The author continues:

"the fastest growing danger of abuse and addiction for the nation's children … came from prescription pills legally manufactured on U.S. soil and sitting in Americans' medicine chest." (p.261)

She points out that there was a convention on psychotropic drugs in 1971 that was signed by dozens of countries to limit the "abuse of addictive psychoactive drugs like barbiturates, amphetamines and LSD. Some of the most frequent violators of the treaty have been companies selling prescription stimulants to American children with attention deficit disorders." (p. 262) Petersen points out that Ritalin contains methylphenidate which she claims "can become a habit if it is misused." (p.262) She writes:" In 2006 researchers estimated that seventy-five thousand teenagers and young adults showed signs of being addicted to stimulants like Concerta, Adderall and Ritalin." (p. 263) There are also reports that grown-ups abused drugs like Ritalin to improve concentration and performance. The author points out that a study in 1987 showed that psychotropic medications like sleeping pills and antidepressants caused more than 32000 elderly Americans to fall and break a hip each year. (p. 300) These drugs can cause dementia or drug induced tremor and can look like the beginning of Parkinson's.) Often the harm is caused by the medication, but the doctor thinks that it is the onset of a new disease. (p.301) She points out that a Canadian study showed that prescription drugs were the fourth leading cause death in the U.S. She feels that autopsies are important to show the effect of dangerous drugs, but that, regrettably, the rate of autopsies has gone down. (p. 309) Petersen points out a disturbing trend: "Inside hospitals and medical offices corporate marketers are now calling the shots. They decide how patients will be treated and the doctors follow along" (p. 321)

Petersen suggests, among others, the following to remedy this situation: (p.324 ff)(I changed the wording of some)

- Families should request autopsies if they wonder about the true cause of death of a loved one. (Medicare pays for that if the person is over 65 years old.)
- The standard death certificate should be redesigned to show if a drug or procedure might have aggravated the patient's condition.
- Doctors should report to MedWatch (FDA) if they suspect that a drug might have caused injury or death.
- Doctors should not be allowed to accept gifts from pharmaceutical companies or have them pay for their education.

- If this is the case, they should let patients know, so they could switch doctors if they so desire.
- Pharmaceutical companies should not be allowed to "ghostwrite" articles in medical publications
- Create a government agency that checks drugs and insist on the agents not having any ties to pharmaceutical companies.
- Tell patients the truth about drugs before they are prescribed and to point out if the prescription is "off-label" and is not approved by the FDA
- Stricter rules for ads should be applied
- Strengthen the FDA
- The pharmaceutical companies should not pay fees for the FDA.
- Celebrities should not be permitted to promote drugs
- "Nonprofit groups should also be prevented from promoting medicines to the public without disclosing they have received money from the drugs manufacturers. Charities should be forced to disclose …how much each company has given them. Some of these groups which pay no taxes, have become…arms of the drug industry" (p.332)
- "Public schools and universities should scrutinize any group offering to educate students about health or screen them for medical problems. The public should also be wary of health fairs or conferences sponsored by the pharmaceutical industry…legislature should question …financial grants the industry gives to state health departments and the agencies that operate the Medicaid program." (p. 332)
- Illegal practices by pharmaceutical companies should be punished.
- Find a doctor who only prescribes pills when necessary and who explains the risk involved.
- Don't take a drug before you know all the risks.
- Be skeptical if a doctor suggests that you take a drug for symptoms that are not actually diseases like prediabetes or prehypertension.
- Contact your state and federal lawmakers and vote for candidates who promise to take on the pharmaceutical industry. (p.335)

Petersen realizes that all drugs have side effects and that often you have to take a drug to get better. But you should carefully weigh the advantages vs. the disadvantages and you should never stop a drug without a doctor's supervision. Finally, Petersen states:

> "By 2007 just about every major pharmaceutical company was under investigation for fraudulent marketing or other illegal business practices.

Prosecutors have tried to discourage the fraud by imposing fines of nearly a billion dollars on some drug companies.

> The pharmaceutical executives appear to consider these fines as little more than a cost of doing business. With no limits on drug prices in America, the companies have simply raised their prices to cover the penalties. Congress must change the law so that pharmaceutical crimes result in harsh penalties for the executives who plan and direct them. Executives should face prison time if they are found to have ordered their employees to engage in illegal practices that put patients' lives at risk." (p. 333)

What role does advertising play in the pharmaceutical industry? The journalist Maggie Mahar writes in her book "Money Driven Medicine "(2006) in regard to advertising: "In 1997 the FDA gave the industry its blessing removing most prohibitions on…advertising. Over the next four years spending on ads…would triple." (p.50) "Up until 1997 the FDA required drug advertisers to provide full information about side effects, making a 30- second spot difficult if not downright frightening. But when it loosened the restrictions, the FDA ruled that drug companies would only have to mention the major risks and refer to…other sources for additional information." (p.365, under notes, no. 68). She continues: "In 2002 drugmakers investing only 19 billion in R &D [and some} 45 billion for marketing, advertising and administration and had a profit of $31 billion" (p.52).

> "In 2002 drug makers laid out over 91 million to support a legion of lobbyists- more than one for every congressperson. (according to Public Citizen Congress Watch 2003) (p.366)

She continues: "In other countries governments regulate prices… (p.286) …with the pipeline of truly innovative drugs drying up, marketing has become the heart of the business."(p.287) "From 1995 to 2002, pharmaceuticals took first prize as the nation's most profitable industry, reporting earnings that ranged from 13 percent to 18.6 percent of sales…every year."(p. 288) She cites Jerry Avorn: "For some large companies paying the drug bills of employees and retirees now consumes fully a quarter of their entire outlay for healthcare."(p. 288)
Maher writes:

> "If the manufacturers and FDA's experts all sit at the same side of the table, no one represents the public's primary need for safety…
> Over the past decade, the FDA's critics claim that the agency has abdicated its role as the public's protector. (p.311)

The agency's priorities started to shift, they suggest, in 1992----when the supposedly independent watchdog agency began to depend on the very companies that it regulates for a major chunk of its funding. That was the year that the pharmaceutical industry finally succeeded in persuading Congress into passing the Prescription Drug User Fee Act (PDUFA)), - a law that aimed to speed up the drug approval process by letting manufacturers fund drug approval."
(p. 311) (s. Angell)

"The 1992 law opened the door to industry funding for faster reviews… Under the original agreement drug makers promised to give the agency 200 million in 1993 – but only if the FDA spent a specified level on new drug approvals. (p.311)
Manufacturers' funding became essential and began to dictate how the FDA spends its money. (p.312) The FDA was forced to shift dollars from other programs to drug approval. In 2003, 79% went to new drug reviews."

> "When doubts about medicines appear, the FDA should insist that drug makers pay for independent tests. If the company refuses the FDA should make that public. Once a drug is approved, doctors and patients assume it's safe. There is no systematic approach to detecting problems after a product goes on the market."

By 2005, the FDA had begun to require post marketing studies of drugs.

Mahar had interviewed Dr. Lazar Greenfield, fellow of the American College of Surgeons and member of many other important medical positions. He said: "Whenever a company feels squeezed, they simply call the congressional people they support – and before long, the congressmen are on the phone to the FDA, saying: 'Back off '." (p.316)

I have always wondered why television and radio channels never seem to be critical of what is happening as a result of the use of psychtropic drugs. In all the suicides, shootings or mass shootings nobody ever seems to ask the question what drug the culprit was taking voluntarily or had to take and why these shootings are happening here and not in other parts of the world. I think I found the answer when I did some research on the money that the pharmaceutical industry spends on advertising. (As you know, the U.S. and New-Zealand are the only two countries in the world that allow this kind of advertising.) I checked the following numbers on Statista (https://www.statista.com.)
<u>Statista</u> wrote on Dec. 20, 2023:
In 2020 TV ad spending of the pharma industry accounted for 75% of the total ad-spending. The numbers were steadily climbing:

In	2016	3.11 billion
	2017	3.45 billion
	2018	3.73 billion
	2019	3.79 billion
	2020	4.58 billion

Attorney Christopher Placitella from the law firm Cohen, Placitella and Roth, who is the firm's lawyer handling medical cases, writes on June 15, 2023:
"Prescription drug advertising is not without its risks." He feels that too much information confuses the patient, even if one side effect is death. He points out that the <u>FDA has an office of Prescription Drug Promotion that warns consumers of the following pitfalls in advertising:</u>

- Omitting or downplaying of risks
- Overstating the drug's benefits
- Failing to present a fair balance of risk and benefit information
- Omitting material facts about the drug

- Making claims that are not appropriately supported
- Misrepresenting data from the studies
- Making misleading drug comparisons
- Misbranding an investigational drug

Of course, I am asking myself how I am supposed to find out the truth about these drugs when the drug companies are not honest about them. I thought this was the role of the FDA. And many people, even educated ones, believe falsely that the FDA checks these drugs before they can be advertised and that the FDA can be trusted.

Everything I have written about the pharmaceutical corporations is extremely negative, because the corporations have adopted Milton Friedman's credo that corporations have no social responsibility, that they are only accountable to the shareholders and that their job is to make as much money for them as possible. I want to cite John C. Bogle, the founder of Vanguard. In his book "Enough" (2009) he expresses an opposing view. He starts out by criticizing the modern corporations. They encourage "...our worship of wealth and the growing corruption of our professional ethics but ultimately the subversion of our character and values." (p.2, 3) He cites economist Henry Kaufman: "Financial institutions and markets must rest on a foundation of trust...Unfettered financial entrepreneurship can become excessive and damaging as well – leading to serious abuses and the trampling of the basic laws and morals of the financial system." (p.69). He writes about medicine:

> "A ...transition has taken place in the medical profession where the human concerns of the caregiver and the human needs of the patient have been overwhelmed by the financial interests of commerce : our giant medical care complex of hospitals, insurance companies, drug manufacturers and marketers and health maintenance organizations..." (p. 125)

And finally, Bogle states about society :

> "It can put honest people on a pedestal even if they do not maximize their personal benefits and preferences...and discard and shun as

models of failure dishonest people who achieve their highest
ambitions by fraud and abuse of trust." (p. 209)

Let us hope that we eventually get to the situation that Bogle wants to achieve.

25. Legal considerations

I recently was told by a friend that her son took his girlfriend to a PCP to get her foot checked. He saw that the doctor had written "mental ?" or something similar on his pad. When I heard this story I wondered what the doctor could or would do with this information. Would this be in her records? He was not a psychiatrist and he had not asked her to fill out a test like e.g. "The depression scale." I pondered questions like: when does a person have to submit to a test, who can order it, and may be, most importantly, does an individual have to take medications even if these are damaging to him?

I have (had) a friend who tried, unsuccessfully, to commit suicide. He survived, but it seems that suicide is considered a mental illness (being seen as part of depression). He had to submit to treatments and medications. The (listed) side effects (increased sex drive) drove him to get involved in an affair which led to his death. Would he not have had the right to refuse the medication on account of its side effects? (The irony is, of course, that many of the psychotropic medications list suicide as side effect!)

I found an article that clarified some aspects in "Everyday Law", Jan. 1989, a publication of Trial Lawyers of America. The author, Michael Szymansky, describes a California case, in which a son almost killed his mother, is serving 12 years in prison, is undergoing psychiatric therapy - but is exercising the right to refuse to take medication ...(the author writes "that might help him")

The author explains that if a mentally ill person commits a minor crime, the police can arrest him and often this person is evaluated. If the person is thought to be mentally ill, he or she can be committed to a psychiatric hospital. He states that every state has a procedure for involuntary civil commitments for people who have not committed a crime. Some states have laws based on a California law which states that nobody can be held against their will unless they are a danger to themselves or others. (of course, I believe it would be easy for a psychiatrist to claim that the person is suicidal.) or if they are "gravely disabled" (which, again, can be easily claimed).The author says: "The involuntary commitment must be determined by a medical doctor, social worker, family member, police officer, court advocate, hearing judge, psychiatrist. In many states the confined can be held against his will from 72 hours to 20 days. He has the right that a regular patient has to know why he is being held, the right to telephone, to visitors, personal possessions and to privacy. The author writes "The right to privacy is so great that most mental institutions will refuse to confirm –even to relatives-that a patient is in their care." He quotes Barbara Demming Lurie, director of the Los Angeles County Mental Patients' Rights Office: "One of the first rights a person should exercise is the right to call an independent advocate." This right was expressed by Congress in the Mental Health Bill of Rights Act with the goal to "establish advocacy and protection in every state." The advocate represents the patient at a hospital hearing where it is determined if the confinement should continue. In most states a new hearing can be scheduled after two weeks to two months. A patient who is not happy with his advocate, can go directly to court to have a judge decide his case. The judge then determines if the patient is a danger to himself or others or is gravely disabled. If the patient answers questions appropriately, he has to be set free. Privacy laws don't allow for inquiry into previous confinement or unusual behavior. The judge must follow state guidelines in this. The guidelines are usually vague like the term dangerous, resulting in "widely diversive decisions." The author further informs us that some states like "Massachussets, New Jersey, New York, Ohio and Oklahoma have allowed patients to refuse treatments-even if they are held against their will-except in emergencies." She continues:

> "Little is known about mental illness, so doctors have to guess at treatments. But most case law suggests patients must give their consent and must be informed of all the side effects of a treatment."

In the case O'Connor v. Donaldson (1975) the Supreme Court ruled that mental illness alone does not justify locking up a person against his will and keeping him locked up. Jim Preis, director of Mental Health Advocacy Services, Inc. maintains "that the mentally ill have the same rights as everyone else."

I recently discussed with a friend the secrecy of personal medical information. He was sure that it was all kept secret. I had come across the Company <u>PharMetrics (s. Peterson , chapter 24)</u> and a statement about it that it kept pharmacy and medical information of 55 million Americans. According to

Wikipedia the company IMS Health acquired PharMetrics in 2005. (accessed on 5.23.2024.)

Adam Tanner wrote in Forbes, Jan. 6, 2014 under the title " Company that knows what Drugs Everyone Takes Going Public":

" Nearly every time you fill out a prescription, your pharmacy sells details of the transaction to outside companies which compile and analyze the information to resell to others. The data includes age and gender of the patient, the name, address and contact details of their doctor, and details about their prescription."

"A 60-year old company, little known by the public, IMS Health is leading the way in gathering this data…IMS Health sells data and reports to all the top 100 worldwide global pharmaceutical and biotechnology companies , as well as consulting firms, advertising agencies, government bodies and finance firms…IMS said it processes data from more (sic) 45 billion healthcare transactions annually …and collects information from more than 780,000 different streams of data worldwide…Pharmaceutical companies want to know what doctors are prescribing what medication… Privacy experts have expressed concern that even anonymized health records, pieced with other information could identify individuals." (IMS stated that that was a risk factor in its business. "Clever outside data scientists" could "unmask" people's identities…"

Bob Merold, a former executive for IMS said that

"the benefits from having this stuff, particular in terms of controlling the health care system and spending is so much greater that we have to live with the risks…"

Deborah Peel, the founder of Patient Privacy Rights in Austin, Texas, "has long been concerned about corporate gathering of medical records." She claims:

"People have been harmed because their records went somewhere they didn't expect…Exponential isn't even a big enough word for how far and how much the data is going to be used in the information age." "Companies dealing in health data must follow the 1996 *Health Insurance Portability and Accountability Act* (HIPPA)…which sets out privacy standards."

IMS statedin its SEC filing: "We continue to engage in strong privacy and security practices in the collection, processing, analysis and use of information."

Addendum I

Abbreviations, laws, organizations, publications and websites:

ABA (American Bar Association-youth at risk) and Youth at RISK
(https://www.americanbar.org/groups/youth at risk.html)

ADR : Adverse drug reaction

Alliance for Human Research Protection (www.ahrp.org): "The aim of this group is
ethical medical research to protect human rights, welfare and dignity"
(Wikipedia))

American Academy of Child and Adolescent Psychiatrists (AACAP): "There have
been concerns about industry-sponsored clinical trials published in the
journal (JAACAP)" (Wikipedia)

American Foundation for Suicide Prevention : Grass root (front group, s.
Addendum)

American Medical Student Association (AMSA): They established "Pharm Free"
project, felt that the medical profession needed more detachment from
pharmaceutical firms, created a Pharm Free Scorecard to evaluate medical
schools according to their pharmaceutical interaction policies. (Wikipedia)

The Annals of Internal Medicine

APA: American Psychiatric Association

Bay-Dole Act: "enabled universities and small businesses to patent discoveries
emanating from research sponsored by the …(NIH) and then to grant
exclusive licenses to drug companies." (Angell)

CDC: Center for Disease Control and Prevention, a government institution

CenterWatch: "company that provides information about the clinical trial
industry." (Angell)

CHADD: Children and Adults with Attention-Deficit /Hyperactivity Disorder (Grass
root (front group) organization

Citizens for better Medicare: Grass root organization, fought "against any kind of
drug price regulation…had ties to big pharma"(Angell, p.201)

CMA (Canadian Medical Association)

CMS (Center for Medicare and Medicaid Services)

Cochran Collaboration: (https://www.chochrane.org)

Corporate Watch: based in the UK. Research group that helps people stand up
against corporations and capitalism.

DEA (Drug Enforcement Administration), a government institution

DrugDex Information Service: established in1997 by Congress, "one of three
organizations that would decide which off-label uses Medicaid would
cover…If a use is listed there, Medicaid must pay…a company with close
connection to the industry…"(Angell,p.204, 205)

DSM (Diagnostic and Statistical Manual of Mental Disorders)

DTC (Direct to consumer advertising)

Eagle Forum: Conservative group stressing family values, founded by Phyllis
Schlafly

Fair balance: Listing risks and benefits of medication equally

False Claim Act: Federal Law to protect against fraudulent (originally war)
profiteers

FDAMA (Food and Drug Administration Modernization Act (1997)): added six
month of patent protection if the drug was tested on children, loosened
"amount of information that must be included in the DTC" (s. Angell)

Foundation for Suicide Prevention

ECRI (EMERGENCY CARE RESEARCH INSTITUTE) (https://home.ecri.org

EIN Presswire (Press release distribution service)
(https://www.einpresswire.com)

GAO (General Accounting Office.)

The Ground Report: (you tube channel)

The Hatch-Waxmann Act: "Expanded monopoly rights (patents) for brand-name
     drugs from eight to fourteen years…" (Angell)

HIPPA (Health Insurance Portability and Accountability Act)

IDEA (Individuals with Disabilities Education Act)-Law that makes free public
     education available for children with disabilities

IMS Health: Company that gathers and sells health information (formerly
     PharMetrics)

INC: (International Control Board)

Jstore (Journalstorage) : not for profit digital library and research platform.
     "provided full text searches for almost 2,000J journals" (Wikipedia)

MEDGUIDE: Digital platform, connects patients, medical professions and
     pharmacists, can track health-related things.

The Medical Whistleblower Advocacy Network (and TEENSCREEN)
     (https://medicalwhistleblower.org>teenscreen)

Medication guide (also referred to as PPI) : Paper included in medication listing
     side effects

Medscape: Online global destination for physicians and healthcare providers
     worldwide, offering the latest medical news. Sister company of WEBMD,

     same criticism as for WebMd: "biasing readers toward drugs." (s. WebMD)

Mental Health Advocacy Services, Inc.

Mental Health Bill of Rights Act, goal "to establish advocacy and protection in
     every state."

MHRA : MEDICINE AND HEALTHCARE PRODUCTS REGULATORY AGENCY (FDA's
     British counterpart)

MTA: (Multimodal treatment study of children with ADHD, sponsored by the
     NIMH.) Often quoted for proving the efficacy of drugs. One investigator

at least had ties to six drug companies. It "…was not placebo-controlled, double-blind clinical study." (Breggin)

NAMI: National Alliance for the Mentally Ill, grass root organization

National Center for Health Statistics (NCHS): US-government agency that provides statistical information. (Wikipedia)

National Council of Juvenile and Family Court Judges

National Depression Awareness Day: Free screening for depression in universities and hospitals

The New American: Right leaning print magazine

NLM (National Library of Medicine), part of the NIH

NIH: (National Institute of Health), a government institution

NIHM: (National Institute of Mental Health), a government institution

NLM: (National Library of Medicine), part of the NIH

NY.Requirements.com

O'Connor v. Donaldson: Supreme Court ruled that mental illness alone does not justify locking up a person against his will and keeping him locked up.

"Off-label (Me too drugs)": "Once… approved it is legal for physicians to prescribe it in any way that they believe is best for the patient."(Petersen)

OIG: Office of Inspector General Bureau of Special Investigations

Open Secrets (https://www.opensecrets.org.) "nonprofit organization that tracks and publishes data on campaign finance and lobbying including a revolving door database which documents the individuals who have worked in both the public sector and lobbying firms and may have conflicts of interest" (Wikipedia, accessed on 7.29.24)

PCORI: (Patient-Centered Outcomes Research Institute (https://www.pcori.org)): independent non-profit research organization created to help patients and those who care for them and partially funded by the government and insurance companies.

PDUFA (Prescription drug user fee): Law aimed to speed drug approval by letting manufacturers fund drug approval .(Angell)

Peter G. Peterson Foundation: Organization dedicated to address economic and fiscal challenges that threaten America's future. (Wikipedia)

PharMetrics (s. IMS) (IMS acquired PharMetrics in2005)

PHRMA: (Pharmaceutical Research and Manufacturers of America). "Main US lobby group" (Angell)

Physician's Desk Reference

PLOS (Public Library of Science) (plos.org) "won't accept pharmaceutical advertisements or pharma-influenced articles "(Wikipedia)

The President's New Freedom Commission on Mental Health: created 2002 by President Bush: "…early screening must become a national goal"(Bush)

PrimeMD: self-help checklist developed by Pfizer (which holds the copyright) to help primary care physicians identify depression. and explains to doctors how to apply for 3rd party reimbursement

PsychDB (Psychiatry Data Base) https://psychdb.com: Created by a Canadian psychiatrist, provides resources for medical students, physicians and residents and tries to be evidence   based.

Psychology Today: Magazine

Psychrights.org

Public Citizen: Advocacy group, started by Ralph Nader

SOCIAL ANXIETY COALITION, advocacy group, sponsored by drug companies (front group)

SSRI (Selective Serotonin Reuptake Inhibitor)

STAT (statnews.com)

Statista (https://www.statista.com)

TEENSCREEN: part of Foundation for Suicide Prevention, terminated in 2012.

United Senior Association: "grass root" i.e. front group, ties to Pharma (Angell)

"U.S. Pharmacist" publication for pharmacists

WebMD : Health information services website. The New York Times wrote:
"biasing readers toward drugs."(2011, by Virginia Heffernan) (Wikipedia)
(s. MEDSCAPE)

WHO (World Health Organization)

wjm: western journal of medicine

Worst pills/best pills (www.worstpills.org.) (part of PublicCitizen) Guide for
medicine

Addendum II

<u>Grass root organizations (front groups) listed by the Citizens'
Commission on Human Rights International (CCHR)</u>

(That means that each group has ties to the pharmaceutical industry
and receives funds from the industry)

- American Foundation for Suicide Prevention
- Anxiety Disorders of America
- Attention Deficit Disorder Association of America
- Center for the Advancement of Children's Mental Health (CACMH)
- Children and Adults with ADD (CHADD)
- Depression and Bipolar Support Alliance (DBSA)
- DBSA Advisory Board
- (Herbert Pardes: Creating the front groups' pipeline)
  (important information)
- Mental Health America (formerly Mental Health Association)
- National Alliance for Mental Illness (NAMI)
- National Association for Research on Schizophrenia and
  Depression (NARSAD)
- Screening for Mental Health Inc.
- Signs of Suicide – Suicide Prevention Action Network USA (SPAN)
- TEENSCREEN- National Center for Mental Health Check checkups
- (TMAP: The Psycho-pharma front business) (important
  information)
- The JED Foundation

What to do:

In regard to

- **Criminal cases and suicides:**   Find out what medication murderers, criminals and suicide victims were using.

  What were the side effects of these medications?

  Consider measure of personal guilt vs. innocence, especially when medication was prescribed without warning of side effects to responsible parts (The Greensburg six or Eric Harris, s. chapter 2)

- **Emil Kraepelin:**   Completely disregard his classification system because of faulty diagnoses (patients were already treated with mind altering drugs as were some of their relatives which led him to his theory of inheriting mental diseases).

  He himself doubted the validity of some of his diagnoses. (He warned of mislabeling)

- **DSM**   Create a panel of members who have no monetary interest in regard to identifying mental disorders, neither now nor in the future. Have them agree on psychiatric diagnosis and terms.

Have medical doctors on the panel who can identify the somatic group of diseases like Premenstrual Syndrome or Post Partum disorder. (These are clearly influenced by hormones)

Don't include disorders that we have not figured out yet, like stuttering.

Include psychologists who are familiar with widely accepted theories, like Freud's "pleasure/ pain principle."

Have some common-sense people, like parents, on the panel who would argue that being sad after the death of a loved one for more than a few months or that fear of public speaking are perfectly normal feeling.

When describing a mental disorder use clear descriptions. One example is the expression "a chemical is thought to be the cause…" used by a government entity. People trust these expressions (after all, they pay for the government.) They should instead say: "It is not clear…"

- ADHD

Needs a total overhaul:
Don't label behaviors that are typical childhood behaviors as a disorder.

Examine the child's background like family, poverty, abuse.

Look at the school situation like block scheduling, poor teaching, not enough time for physical exercise.

Be aware of parents who take advantage of government support when they identify their children with ADHD. (as described by Bruce Levine) Use talk therapy before you put your child on medication

Have health care provider and parent sign a paper that warns of the side effects of the medication. Make sure that the dosis is correct and make sure that several psychiatric drugs are not prescribed together. (The same applies to children in foster care, the prison population, veterans, older people in homes and the homeless.)

- Medical:

Don't allow suppression of negative results-have <u>all</u> results published.

Demand that pharmaceutical firms test the success of drug and test the drugs for a longer (set) period of time

Find psychiatrist and psychologists
who practice alternative methods
(i.e. drugfree methods) to deal
with mental problems.

- Financial background

Make government jobs honorary. (A
pipe dream) (s. above)
(The author Edith Hamilton felt that
Greece lost its freedom and integrity
once she started to pay her
representatives.)

Don't allow lobbying or political
contribution by pharmaceutical
companies.
Don't allow politicians to get a job
with these companies in the future.

Since taxpayers pay for the research,
let them partake in the profit instead
of giving it to the companies.

Change corporations-that means
more government oversight.
Corporations should not be allowed
to make profit their only goal-to the
detriment of the population. (Milton
Friedman's view vs. John Bogle's.)

Provide more scrutiny for off-
label drugs

Don't allow mixture of public
Interest groups and corporations
like CHADD or NAMI. The public is

often not aware that corporations are behind these groups.

Don't allow gun sales to people who use psychotropic drugs.

- What we can do:

We can use a petition and have it signed by friends and neighbors. It would be worth the effort to avoid sad and senseless killings and suicides.

Epilogue

Psychotropic drugs are used to treat mental disorders. The definition of these disorders are based on an outdated system by a doctor, Emil Kraepelin, who himself based his definitions largely on the examination of people who had been treated with drugs that caused mental disabilities (like Mercury). Pharmaceutical companies have a huge impact on the definitions (and make a lot of money in the process.) These mental disorders are, to a great extent, normal human behavior (like over-eating, sadness after a death, anxiety, fear of public speaking.) When more than half of the population has these behaviors, they are average and should not be labelled as mental disorder. These disorders also show that they have not been influenced by the knowledge that philosophers, psychiatrists, psychologists etc. have accumulated over time. Psychotropic drugs can be used "off-label" and by regular doctors –a very dangerous practice. As faulty as these definitions are as powerful they are legally –they can deprive people of their legal rights or force them to take disabling drugs. Many people in important positions are unaware of the dangers that these drugs represent. They are often prescribed for a much longer time than they have been tested for and they can cause psychotic behavior rather than cure it thus entangling the patient in a web that may leave him much worse off than before.

It is easy to be confused about psychotropic drugs. Many of us are nervous about our children becoming depressed or not doing well in school. The advice we get is often not based on solid scientific knowledge. We tend to trust what the FDA or the NIMH recommend, not knowing that they are, to a great extent, intertwined with the corporations (although they are paid with our tax dollars.) Unfortunately, many politicians are, too. (Citizens United doesn't help!)

We, the taxpayers, work every day to pay for our representatives to help and protect us. This is not always the case. Our tax dollars also pay for research that is then used by the corporations for profit and for the FDA supposedly being a watchdog for medications and yet we pay exorbitant prices (the highest in the world!) for our medications while the corporations get many tax breaks. Often, international companies can sell medication here that they are not allowed to sell in their own country.

What can we do? Get trustworthy information from the Internet ("consider the source!") and, if you can find it in your heart, circulate the petition.

Let's hope that we can change the laws to protect our loved ones.

Bibliography

Angell, Marcia : "The Truth about the Drug Companies", Random House, Trade paperback edition, 2005

Bakan, Joel: "The Corporation. The Pathological Pursuit of Profit and Power", Viking, Canada, 2004

"Childhood under Siege – how Big Business Targets Children", First Free Press hardcover 2011

Belzer, Richard and Wayne, David: "Corporate Conspiracies. How Wall Street took over Washington", Skyhorse Publishing, 2017

Bogle, John: "Enough. True Measures of Money, Business and Life", John Wiley and Sons, Inc. 2009

Breggin, Peter:

"Toxic Psychiatry", St. Martin's Press, 1991

"Talking Back to Prozac. What Doctors won't tell you about today's most Controversial Drug, St. Martin's Press, 1995

Breggin, Peter and Cohen, David: "Your Drug may be your Problem", Perseus Books, Reading Mass. 1999

Breggin, Peter:" Talking back to Ritalin", 2011

Caplan, Paula: "They Say You're crazy – How the World's Most Powerful Psychiatrists Decide who is normal", Addison-Wesley Publishing Company 1995

Conrad, Peter: "The Medicalization of Society", Johns Hopkins University Press, 2007

Glenmullen, Joseph: "Prozac Backlash", Simon and Schuster, 2000

Goldacre, Ben: "Bad Pharma – How Drug Companies mislead doctors and harm patients", Faber and Faber, 2012

Greenberg, Gary: "Manufacturing Depression – the Secret History of a Modern Disease", Simon and Schuster, 2010

Greenberg, Gary: "The Book of Woe", Plume, Penguin Group, 2013

Greenspan, Stanley: "Overcoming ADHD", Da Capo Press, 2009

Hamilton, Edith: "The Echo of Greece", W.W. Norton and Company Inc., New York, 1957

Horwitz, Allan and Wakefield, Jerome: "The Loss of Sadness. How Psychiatry Transformed Normal Sorrow into Depressive Disorder", Oxford University Press, 2007

Hughes, Richard and Brewin, Robert: " The Tranquilizing of America – Pill Popping and the American Way of Life", Harcourt, Brace, Jovanovich, Inc.1979

Kirk, Stuart A. and Kutchins, Herb: "Making us Crazy", the Free Press, 1997

"The Selling of DSM", New Paperback Printing, 2008, Transaction Publishers, New Brunswick, N.J.

Kraepelin, Emil: "Lectures on Clinical Psychiatry" Special Edition, 1988. The Classics of Psychiatry and Behavioral Sciences Library, Division of Gryphon Editions, Inc., PO Box 76108, Birmingham, Ala. 35253

Levine, Bruce E.: "A Profession without Reason-the Crisis of Contemporary Psychiatry Untangled and Solved by Spinoza, Freethinking and Radical Enlightment", AK Press 2022

Mahar, Maggie: "Money Driven Medicine", Harper Collins, 2006

McGoey , Linsey: "No Such Thing as a Free Gift – the Gates Foundation and the Price of Philantrophy", Verso, 2016.

Mayes, Rick, Bagwell, Catherine and Erkulwater, Jennifer: "Medicating Children", Harvard University Press, 2009

Mendelsohn, Robert: "How to Raise a Healthy Child in spite of your Doctor", Ballantine books, 1987

Moncrieff, Joanna: "A Straight Talking Introduction to Psychiatric Drugs", 2nd edition, PCCS books, 2020

Moynihan, Ray and Cassels, Alan: "Selling Sickness", Nation Books, 2005

Northrup, Christiane : "The Wisdom of Menopause", Bantam revised edition, 2006

Pert, Candace: "Molecules of Emotions", Simon and Schuster, 1997

Peterson, Melody: "Our Daily Meds", Sarah Crichton Books, Farrar, Straus and Giroux, 2008

Posner, Gerald: " Pharma –Greed, Lies and the Poisoning of America", Avid Reader Press, 2020

Richter, Franz: "Wir leben chemisch", Verlag für Jugend und Volk, 1967

Tone, Andrea: "The Age of Anxiety", Basic Books, 2009

Wohl, Stanley: "The Medical Industrial Complex, Harmony Books, N.Y. 1984

*Please copy the following pages, (double sided), staple and distribute them with your petition.

(The courts accept FDA statements, so it is especially important for them to familiarize themselves with the following statements.)

PSYCHOTROPIC MEDICATION

Warnings by FDA, DEA, NIH and UN
(https://www.accessdata.fda.gov.>drugsatfda docs.)

The most important facts about psychotropic drugs (s. Chapter13):

There are:

Antidepressants: (e.g. Luvox, Prozac, Zoloft)

antipsychotic agents: (e.g. Haldol, Risperdal, Seroquel, Zyprexa)

stimulants (amphetamines):   (e.g. Adderall, Dexetrine, Effexor, Ritalin)

anti-anxiety agents: (e.g. Cymbalta, Librium, Valium)

sedatives: (e.g. Amytal)

The Food and Drug Administration published the following warnings in the following article:

Suicidality in children and Adolescents Being treated with **Antidepressant Medication**

On February 5, the FDA directed all manufacturers of all antidepressants to revise their labelling by adding a boxed warning and extended warning statements to alert health care providers to an increased risk of suicidal thinking and behavior in children and adolescents who are treated with these antidepressants and to include information about pediatric studies. The FDA has informed the manufacturers that it decided that a Med Guide (Patient Medication Guide) will be given to each patient who takes these drugs to advise them of risks and precautions they may want to take.

These labelling changes were made after recommendations by the Psychopharmacologic Drugs Advisory Committee and the Pediatric Drugs Advisory Committee on September 13-14, 2004.
The risks of suicidality were identified in placebo-controlled trials that lasted 4 months. Nine drugs were examined, including the SSRIs which were prescribed for children and adolescents with psychiatric disorders. There were 24 trials involving 4400 patients. The risk for suicidality for patients on these drugs was 4%, vs. placebo risk of 2% (No suicides occurred during the testing.) The FDA decided to include the following points in the boxed warnings:

- Risk of suicidality
- For clinical use this risk must be balanced with the clinical need.
- Patients on these medications should be observed for this risk, for clinical worsening or unusual changes in behavior.
- Families and caregivers should closely observe the patient and communicate with the prescriber.
- A statement as to whether a drug is approved for any pediatric use and if so, which one.

Pediatric patients should be closely observed for clinical worsening, agitation, irritability, suicidality and unusual changes in behavior or at times of dose changes.

The FDA has included the following drugs that should include these warnings:

Anafranil	Paxil
Aventyl	Pexeva
Celexa	Prozac
Cymbalta	Remeron
Desyrel	Sarafem
Effexor	Serzone
Elavyl	Sinequan
Lexapro	Surmontil
Limbitrol	Symbiax
Ludiomil	Tofranil

Luvox   Tofranil PM
Marplan   Triavil
Nardil   Norpramin
Vivactil   Wellbutrin
Pamelo   Zoloft
Parnate   Zyban

On its website the **FDA** <u>warns of side effects of</u> **stimulants** <u>(website, see above):</u>

> "patients being considered for treatment should have a thorough examination for <u>heart related diseases</u> in themselves or their family…Patients who develop symptoms …of cardiac disease during stimulant treatment should undergo a prompt cardiac evaluation."

> <u>Psychiatric Adverse Events:</u> The FDA warns that "stimulants may exacerbate symptoms in "patients with preexisting psychotic disorders…" but also <u>warns of new psychotic or manic symptoms:</u>

> <u>Emergence of New Psychotic or Manic Symptoms:</u>
> "…psychotic or manic symptoms, e.g. hallucinations, delusional thinking or mania in children or adolescents <u>without prior history of psychotic</u> <u>illness…can be caused by stimulants at usual doses</u>. IF SUCH SYMPTOMS OCCUR, CONSIDERATION SHOULD BE GIVEN TO A POSSIBLE CAUSAL ROLE IN THE STIMULANT, and discontinuation of treatment may be appropriate."

The following are more detailed **<u>warnings by the FDA:</u>**

<u>Aggression:</u> "Aggressive behavior or hostility is often observed in children and adolescents with ADHD and has been reported in clinical trials and the post marketing experience of some medications indicated for the treatment of ADHD…patients beginning treatment for ADHD should be monitored for the <u>appearance of or worsening of</u> <u>aggressive behavior or hostility."</u>

 Long-Term Suppression of Growth: There is a suggestion "that consistently
medicated children have a temporary slowing in growth rate without
evidence of rebound during this period of development… therefore
patients who are not growing or gaining weight as expected may
need to have their treatment interrupted."

Seizures: "There is some clinical evidence that stimulants may lower the
convulsive threshold…very rarely, in patients without a history of
seizures…In the presence of seizures the drug should be
discontinued.

Peripheral Vasculopathy, Including Raynaud's Phenomenon: "Stimulants,
including Adderall, used to treat ADHD are associated with [these
diseases]…very rare sequelae included digital ulceration and/or soft
tissue breakdown…Careful observation for digital changes is
necessary. Effects [of the above diseases] were observed …at
therapeutic doses in all age groups…Careful observation for digital
changes is necessary…Further clinical observation (e.g.,
rheumatology referral) may be appropriate for certain patients."

Serotonin Syndrome basically happens when there is too much
serotonin in the body (this can happen because the reuptake that
occurs naturally, is inhibited by medication, the SSRIs, because of a
combination with other SSRIs. The FDA : [This is]"a potentially life-
threatening reaction … In these situations, consider an alternative to
non-serotonergic drug…Serotonin syndrome symptoms may include
mental status changes instability (e.g. tachycardia, labile blood
pressure, dizziness, diaphoresis, flushing, hyperthermia),
neuromuscular symptoms (e.g. agitation, hallucinations, delirium and
coma, autonomic tremor, rigidity, myoclonus, hyperreflexia,
incoordination), seizures, and/or gastrointestinal symptoms (e.g.,
nausea, vomiting, diarrhea)"

<u>Visual Disturbances</u>: "Difficulties with accommodation and blurring of vision have been reported with <u>stimulant</u> treatment"

<u>Tics:</u>   "<u>Amphetamines</u> have been reported to <u>exacerbate motor and phonic tics and Tourette's syndrome</u>... clinical evaluation [for these] should precede use of stimulant medication."

The FDA adds the following:
<u>Information for patients:</u>
" Prescribers or other health professionals should inform patients, their families and their caregivers about the benefits and <u>risks associated with treatment with amphetamine or dextroamphetamines</u> and should counsel them in its appropriate use. A patient Medication Guide is available for Adderall."
The FDA urges health professionals to instruct patients, their families and caregivers to discuss the contents of this guide and to obtain answers.

And what does the **<u>DEA</u>** (Department of Justice/United States Drug Enforcement Administration), a government entity, say about **amphetamines (stimulants)**? <u>(under drug fact sheet):</u>

"What is their effect on the body? Similar to cocaine, but slower onset and longer duration, increased body temperature, blood pressure and pulse, insomnia, loss of appetite, physical exhaustion. <u>Chronic abuse produces a psychosis that resembles</u> <u>schizophrenia: paranoia, hallucinations, violent and erratic behavior.</u>

What does the **NIH** (National Institute of Health), a U.S. Government entity, say about the effects of **sedatives?**

Short term symptoms of use:
Drowsiness
Sedation
<u>slurred speech</u>

Poor concentration

Confusion

Dizziness

Clammy skin

Impaired judgment, coordination and memory

Reduced anxiety (?)

Lowered blood pressure

Slowed breathing

They name, among others: Nembutal, Luminal, Xanax, Limbitrol, Valium, Ativan, Halicon, Lunesta, Sonata, Ambien.

The **DEA** (United States Drug Enforcement Administration) lists 5 groups of substances (schedules) that are essential for law enforcement. Let's look at Schedule II.

Schedule II: Drugs with a high potential for abuse [and] … and psychological and physical dependence. These drugs are also considered dangerous. (e.g. Methamphetamine, Methadone, Demerol, Dexedrine, Adderall, Ritalin.

Let's take a look at the warning the **FDA** issues for some well known psychotropic medications (https://www.accessdata.fda.gov.>drugsatfda docs.) As of March 2012) Most of them are stimulants (amphetamines) The FDA approves some of them starting at the age 3-6 years, most at the age of 6 years, but also includes the following warnings (side effects):

Celexa (Citalopram)   Is an SSRI, can be fatal, should be avoided. "In 3 additional placebo controlled in depressed patients…the difference between patients receiving Celexa and patients receiving a placebo was not statistically different."

Effexor   Can cause mania, suicidal thinking.

Luvox:	Side effects: Anxiety, agitation, panic attacks…, irritability, hostility, aggressiveness, psychomotor restlessness
	Can cause, among others, anxiety, agitation, panic attacks, hostility, aggression, increase in suicidal thinking
Prozac	SSRI
	Side effects: Mania, seizures, anxiety, potential for cognitive and motor impairment, suicidal thoughts and behavior. Can cause serotonin syndrome when used with other serotonergic agents (other antidepressants or herbs.)
Ritalin	SSRI
	Suitable for pediatric patients 6 years and older
	Side effects: Serious cardiovascular events, may cause psychotic or manic symptoms in patients with no prior history of symptoms like hallucinations and delusional thinking, painful prolonged penile erection, long-term suppression of growth, anxiety, insomnia, abdominal pain
Seroquel	for bipolar disorder, efficacy was established in 2 twelve week monotherapy trials
	Side effects: Suicidal thoughts or behavior, tardive dyskinesia, potential for cognitive and motor impairment, abnormal thinking (p.27).
Xanax	Antianxiety
	Side effects: Seizures after withdrawal, mania, suicide
Zoloft	SSRI, for, among others, PTSD
	Side effects: Suicidal thoughts and behavior, difficulty concentrating, confusion, unsteadiness

I also want to include again the warnings by the <u>United Nations about Ritalin</u> that I mentioned in chapter 15.

In 1995 (released in 1996) the **United Nations** released the following warning in regard to Ritalin:

> the <u>United Nation</u>, in its annual report, the UN's International Narcotics Control Board, issued a warning about <u>Ritalin</u> (Methylphenidate) under the title "Dramatic Increase in Methylphenidate Consumption in US: Marketing Methods Questioned". The report states that the drug was classified as a schedule II drug as having high abuse potential. The international Narcotics Control Board has observed a world use of Methylphenidate rose from 3 tonnes in 1990 to more than 8.5 tonnes in 1994, and continued to rise. The United States accounts for about 90 percent of total world manufacture and consumption. The ...sharp increase is due to its controversially extensive use in the treatment of ADD (now called ADHD) in children. The INCB shares its concern with the US Drug Enforcement Agency (DEA) The danger the Board sees is overpresciption. Also, the duration of treatment is restricted in many countries to three years, it tends to be much longer in the US... many children remain on it into adolescence, even adulthood although there are no tests that examine the side effects of such long-term treatment.
> There is an increase of abuse of Ritalin with serious damage to health like addiction and stimulant –abuse symptoms.
> "The INCB is also concerned that the use of Ritalin is being actively promoted by an influential parent association which has received significant contribution from the "the US manufacturer of the drug.
> "This association has petitioned the DEA to ease the control ..."
> "At the present, the unprecedented high level of ADD [ADHD] in children, the very widespread prescription of Ritalin and the growing abuse and black market appear to be limited to the United States" The board sees a danger that these problems will take hold

**in other countries and states that some of the parent groups
indicated that they will promote the use in other countries.
"The Board is therefore requesting all governments to exercise
utmost vigilance to prevent the overdiagnosing of ADD and any
medically-unjustified treatment with Methylphenidate and other
stimulants. It has also requested the World Health Organization
(WHO) to investigate this matter and to provide expertise to
national public health authorities."**

The report adds the following:

**"...Concern has been raised that doctors are resorting to
Methylphenidate as an "easy" solution for behavioral problems
which may have complex causes. Critics warn that parents' and
teachers' assessments of what constitutes "inattention" and
"impulsivity" are highly subjective and that doctors prescribing
practices for Methylphenidate are far from uniform."**

(Source: QWQED-FRONTLINE)

How to handle petition

- Please copy the previous pages with the warnings by the FDA, DEA, NIH and UN. Please cut out petition and make copies.

- Explain background and reason for the petition.

- Ask person (neighbor, friend, acquaintance, to also get involved.

- Send pages and petitions (or call) your representative.

Thank you!

(We petition our lawmakers to make a law requesting the prescriber and patient to fill out this sheet before each prescription)

Petition

(This should be filled out by prescriber and patient)

*   I, the prescriber……………………………. have pointed out to the patient and
*   his/her caregiver the side-effects of the drug_______________________________
*   which are the following:

*

*   ____

*

*   ____

*

*   --

*

*   ____

*

*   I have enclosed the FDA, DEA and United Nations' warning.

*

*   I will further monitor the dosage and duration of this medication and
*   its effect on this patient.

*

*   I will not allow the off-label prescription or combination with other drugs *
    without a secondary review.

*

*   Alternative therapies should be used before and at the same time of

*   administration of this drug.

*   (* partially based on American academy of child and adolescent psychiatry.)

*

*   Signed by prescriber:____

    Signed by patient or caregiver:_______________________________

hmm6@pitt.edu

www.ingramcontent.com/pod-product-compliance
Lightning Source LLC
Chambersburg PA
CBHW081209260726
48653CB00010BA/3579